CASE REVIEW
Musculoskeletal Imaging

Series Editor
David M. Yousem, MD
Professor, Department of Radiology
Director of Neuroradiology
Johns Hopkins Hospital
Baltimore, Maryland

Other Volumes in the CASE REVIEW Series
Brain Imaging
Breast Imaging
Cardiac Imaging
Gastrointestinal Imaging
General and Vascular Ultrasound
Genitourinary Imaging
Head and Neck Imaging
Nuclear Medicine
OB/GYN Ultrasound
Pediatric Imaging
Thoracic Imaging
Vascular and Interventional Imaging

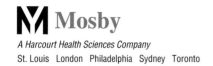

Mosby

A Harcourt Health Sciences Company

St. Louis London Philadelphia Sydney Toronto

Joseph Yu, MD
Associate Professor of Radiology
Ohio State University College of Medicine
Chief of Musculoskeletal Imaging
Ohio State University Medical Center
Program Director, Diagnostic
Radiology Residency
Ohio State University Medical Center
Columbus, Ohio

CASE REVIEW

Musculoskeletal Imaging

CASE REVIEW SERIES

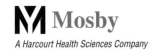

Mosby
A Harcourt Health Sciences Company

Acquisitions Editor: Stephanie Donley
Project Manager: Agnes Byrne
Manuscript Editor: Jennifer Ehlers
Senior Production Manager: Peter Faber
Illustration Specialist: Lisa Lambert
Book Designer: Gene Harris
Cover Designer: Catherine Bradish

Mosby, Inc.
A Harcourt Health Sciences Company

11830 Westline Industrial Drive
St. Louis, Missouri 63146

Printed in the United States of America

Library of Congress Cataloging-in-Publication Data

Yu, Joseph.

Musculoskeletal imaging: case review/Joseph Yu.

p. cm.

ISBN 0–323–01620–0

1. Musculoskeletal system—Imaging—Case studies. I. Title.

RC925.7.Y8 2002

616.7'0754—dc21   2001034568

00 01 02 03 04/9 8 7 6 5 4 3 2 1

To Cindy for her unyielding love and understanding, to Sarah for helping me to view things with an enthusiastic and interested perspective, to Jim and John for their support, and to Mom and Dad, who remain my source of inspiration.

The Case Review Series is designed to review each specialty in a challenging, interactive way. Each book in the series has gradations of difficulty so that the reader can assess his or her proficiency and can use this self-evaluation to guide continued education. Because each case in the book is distinct, this is the kind of text that can be picked up and read at any time in your day, in your career.

When I had a choice of whom to select to write *Musculoskeletal Imaging: Case Review*, I had several criteria. The person must be a leading authority in the field, a great teacher, enthusiastic, conscientious, and a disciple of Don Resnick. Joe Yu fit the bill entirely, and, of all the authors solicited for this series, he has been the most energetic and enthusiastic. I think that you can get a sense of those traits in his book. This is a great contribution to the teaching field. Dr. Yu has selected an outstanding array of cases and modalities that teach musculoskeletal imaging. The accompanying text includes many references as well as tricks of the trade to guide the practitioner.

I am very pleased to have Dr. Yu's edition join the ever-expanding Case Review Series. I welcome *Musculoskeletal Imaging: Case Review* to the others in our series: *Obstetrical and Gynecologic Ultrasound* by Al Kurtz and Pam Johnson; *Thoracic Imaging* by Phil Boiselle and Theresa McLoud; *Genitourinary Imaging* by Glenn Tung, Ron Zagoria, and William Mayo-Smith; *Gastrointestinal Imaging* by Peter Feczko and Robert Halpert; *Brain Imaging* by Laurie Loevner; and *Head and Neck Imaging* by myself. Congratulations to Dr. Yu for a job well done.

David M. Yousem, MD
Case Review Series Editor

One of the most difficult challenges in life is discovering the things that motivate you and help keep you going. We are faced with this dilemma in nearly every facet of our daily lives, whether it is professionally or at home.

Education is one of my passions. Early in my medical training, I discovered that teaching fulfilled me, and it was at that time that I decided to set a career path in academia. Nearly a decade has passed, and I find myself undaunted by the constant renewing of residents going through our program and by taking them from neophyte clinicians to competent radiologists. I find myself refreshed and rejuvenated by the enthusiasm and inquisitive nature of those by whom I am surrounded, and it is this curiosity that keeps me motivated to maintain a constant vigilance for updated information to pass on.

I am thankful to have the opportunity to contribute to the Case Review Series. I like the format provided in this series because it engages the reader to commit to a diagnosis or to formulate a list of differential possibilities before the answer is divulged. Not meant to be a comprehensive text, it still allows emphasis of important concepts regarding the entity covered in each case. The questions are meant to simulate those that one may encounter in an examination. In keeping with Dr. Yousem's theme, I have not cited articles that are necessarily "classics" in musculoskeletal imaging but have emphasized more recent literature. I have chosen representative cases from different areas of osteoradiology and have made an attempt to include as many imaging modalities as possible, with one notable exception—ultrasound. I admit that we rarely perform sonography for musculoskeletal conditions in my institution, so I have little experience with and even less access to such cases.

I want to thank Dr. Donald Resnick, a teacher and colleague who continues to inspire me to reach for new heights. Under the tutelage of Dr. Resnick and his partners, Dr. Mini Pathria and the late Dr. David Sartoris, I gained valuable experience in both teaching and learning. I want to thank Dr. Javier Beltran for instilling in me the desire to become just like him, an accomplished osteoradiologist, when I was a second-year resident. I want to thank my partners, Drs. Carol Ashman and Marcella Dardani, for helping me compile an excellent teaching file from which to draw my cases for this book. I especially want to thank all residents and fellows, past and present, for nurturing my need to teach and responding favorably to my style of teaching.

I also would like to thank my chairman, Dr. Dimitrios Spigos, and all my colleagues for their support. I want to thank Liz Corra of Mosby and Stephanie Donley of Harcourt Health Sciences for their excellent editorial management. I want to thank Nydic Open MRI of Cleveland, Boardman, and Kettering for providing me with many of the cases shown in this book and for continuing to keep my teaching file well stocked. And to Theron Ellinger and John Croyle for their excellent photographic support, and to Sandy Baker for her secretarial assistance, goes my gratitude.

Most of all, I want to thank Cindy, my wife, for enduring my idiosyncrasies during this past year and for helping and encouraging me to finish despite many distractions. And lastly, to the jewel of my life, my daughter Sarah, thanks for your understanding during the times that I could not play with you.

Joseph Yu, MD

Opening Round

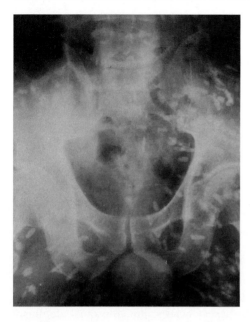 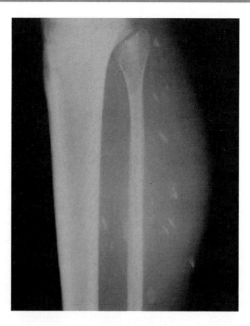

1. What is the parasite responsible for this condition? How do humans become infected?
2. Where does the adult worm reside in the human body?
3. What is the appearance of the scolex, one of the parasite's identification markers?
4. Is there any blood test that is diagnostic for this disease?

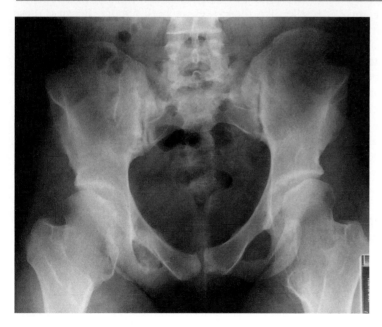

1. What is the diagnosis?
2. What are some potential complications seen in patients with this disorder?
3. A painful growth spurt of a lesion in a skeletally mature patient may be indicative of what condition?
4. Define Trevor's disease.

C A S E 1

Cysticercosis

1. The larval form of *Taenia solium*. By ingestion of infested pork that has been incompletely cooked.

2. In the upper jejunum.

3. Two rows of hooklets.

4. No, indirect hemagglutination is the best serologic test available.

Reference

Reeder MM: Tropical diseases of the soft tissues. Semin Roentgenol 8:47-71, 1973.

Comments

The key to diagnosis in this case is the appearance of each calcification and the widely scattered distribution. This patient from Mexico presented with symptoms of meningoencephalitis. Human tapeworms require one or more intermediate hosts for larval development. Ingestion of tissues that contain cysts with viable scolices by a definitive host allows maturation of the larval stage of a worm into its adult form. *Taenia solium* is a unique parasite because humans may act as both its definitive and its intermediate hosts. Invasion of human tissue by the larval form is the disease termed *cysticercosis.* Infection is caused by consumption of infected pork. Once the parasite is in the body, humans may become autoinfected when gravid segments of the worm are returned to the stomach by reverse peristalsis. The infected human also acts as an intermediate host, because the embryo released from the egg penetrates the intestinal wall and is then dispersed to other parts of the body through the blood stream. The larval form becomes encysted in the muscles, subcutaneous tissues, viscera, heart, eye, and brain (cerebrum, ventricles, subarachnoid space), and the clinical manifestation of the disease occurs in response to the larvae once it has died. Note the characteristic "ricelike" calcifications diffusely scattered in the striated muscles. Muscular pain, weakness, fever, and eosinophilia were pertinent findings in this patient. The differential list is small. *Loa loa* infestation may have a similar appearance but is seldom as extensive and is localized primarily to the subcutaneous tissues.

C A S E 2

Hereditary Multiple Exostosis

1. Hereditary multiple exostosis (HME).

2. Impairment of joint function, reactive bursal formation, and mechanical pressure on adjacent neurovascular structures or spinal cord.

3. Malignant transformation.

4. Exostoses involving the epiphyses (dysplasia epiphysealis hemimelica).

Reference

Black B, Dooley J, Pyper A, Reed M: Multiple hereditary exostoses. An epidemiologic study of an isolated community in Manitoba. Clin Orthop 287:212-217, 1993.

Comments

This patient demonstrates classic findings of HME, also known as diaphyseal aclasis, an autosomal dominant metaphyseal hyperplastic disorder characterized by the development of multiple osteochondromas. Most patients present with a discovery of a single or multiple painless masses near the joints, usually in the first decade of life. The lesions typically form and enlarge during growth until the skeleton is fully matured. Although some osteochondromas are pedunculated (note lesion in the right side of pubis), most are broad based and sessile, like those seen in both femora. Because these osteochondromas frequently involve a large circumference of the metaphyseal region, this condition can mimic a bone dysplasia. Diminished tubulation of the ends of the long bones often results in a broadened shaft; hence the term diaphyseal aclasis. When the lower extremities are asymmetrically affected, compensatory scoliosis can occur. A family history is identified in 70% of cases. Each patient may have anywhere from a few to several hundred lesions.

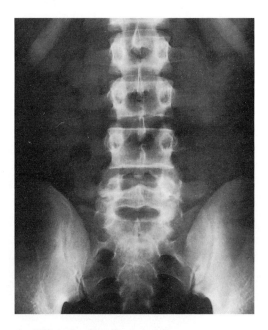 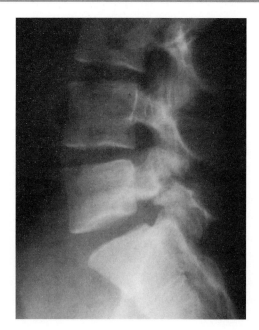

1. What is the diagnosis?
2. List several proposed causes for this condition.
3. What do you look for on computed tomography (CT) scan?
4. If the process is unilateral, what are some associated radiographic findings?

Spondylolysis

1. Spondylolysis of L5.

2. The cause of spondylolysis is controversial: both congenital (hypoplasia or aplasia) and acquired (pseudoarthrosis secondary to fracture from repeated trauma or underlying bone disease) theories have been proposed.

3. (1) Located approximately 10 to 15 mm above the disk level, (2) having an irregular noncorticated margin, (3) located anterior to the facet joint and oriented in a more coronal plane, and (4) with an intact cortical ring around the spinal canal.

4. Contralateral neural arch sclerosis and hypertrophy.

Reference

Grogan JP, Hemminghytt S, Williams AL, et al: Spondylolysis studied with computed tomography. Radiology 145:737–742, 1982.

Comments

Spondylolysis refers to a defect through the pars interarticularis of a vertebra. The pars interarticularis bridges the superior and inferior articular processes, depicted by uninterrupted cortices and continuous bone marrow. In patients with spondylolysis, an obliquely oriented cleft bisects the pars. The incidence of spondylolysis increases with age and has been estimated to be about 5% in the general population. Among patients with low back pain, however, the incidence may be as high as 10%. The L5 vertebra is the most common location for spondylolysis, followed in incidence by the L4 vertebra. These two levels account for 90% of all spondylolytic defects. When the defect is bilateral, it can be associated with spondylolisthesis. The most widely accepted theory for its development is repeated minor trauma causing a break in the pars interarticularis, much like a stress fracture. The diagnosis using CT can be challenging. Spondylolysis may resemble a facet joint but with several differences as listed previously. Recall that a facet joint is located at the level of the disk, is oriented obliquely, and contains smooth cortical margins. Callus formation or granulation tissue adjacent to a pars defect is present in about 20% of cases and may indicate instability. Single photon emission computed tomography (SPECT) scintigraphy is useful to determine metabolic activity, because compression of a nerve root can be a potential complication.

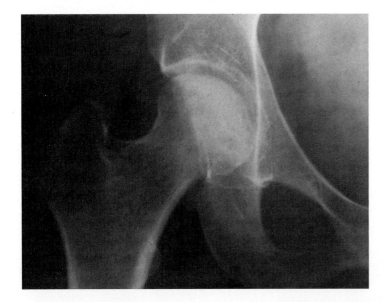
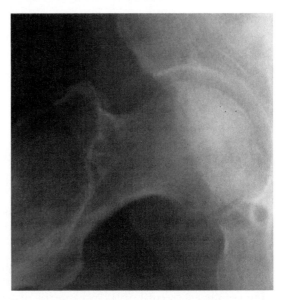

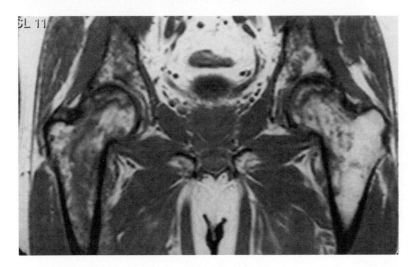

1. Name Ficat's stages of osteonecrosis.

2. Is the presence of bone marrow edema on magnetic resonance imaging (MRI) always indicative of avascular necrosis?

3. What histopathologic factors contribute to the development of avascular necrosis?

4. What are the causes of posttraumatic avascular necrosis of the femoral head?

Femoral Head Avascular Necrosis

1. In Ficat's classification, stage 1 is normal, or slightly increased or diminished density; stage 2 is mixed osteopenia and sclerosis; stage 3 is subchondral collapse or a "crescent" sign; stage 4 is articular collapse; and stage 5 is progression to degenerative joint disease.

2. No, it may also be seen in transient osteoporosis of the hip, transient bone marrow edema syndrome, infection, trauma, and neoplasms.

3. (1) Thrombosis, embolism, or disruption of vascular supply of femoral head and (2) weakening of the bone marrow from repetitive exposure to cytotoxic factors.

4. Poor alignment; unstable reduction; and disruption of the femoral circumflex (medial or lateral) arteries, the epiphyseal (medial or lateral) arteries, or both.

Reference

Gillespy T 3rd, Genant HK, Helms CA: Magnetic resonance imaging of osteonecrosis. Radiol Clin North Am 24:193–208, 1986.

Comments

Avascular necrosis indicates bone death, most commonly owing to ischemia. Etiologic factors that contribute to the development of avascular necrosis of the femoral head include trauma, hematologic conditions (systemic lupus erythematosus, Gaucher's disease), Cushing's syndrome or exogenous corticosteroid administration, alcoholism, pancreatitis, pregnancy, and Caisson's disease. MRI has proven to be very efficacious in assessing patients with hip pain and risk factors for developing avascular necrosis. Direct visualization of the bone marrow enables detection at an earlier stage than is allowed with conventional radiography. In the acute phase of the disease, bone marrow edema involving the femoral head may be the only notable finding. In the absence of any risk factors, osteonecrosis is only one of a number of other potential diagnoses. If the ischemic process worsens, a "double line" sign becomes evident, a characteristic finding in advanced avascular necrosis. This sign, an irregular rim of low signal intensity on T1W images and paired rims of high and low signal intensities on T2W images, identifies the interface between viable and dying bone marrow. The high signal intensity rim is indicative of granulation tissue, and the adjacent low signal intensity rim reflects cellular debris, fibrous tissue, and reactive trabecular bone.

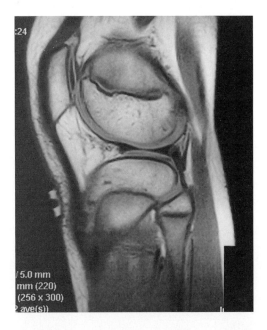

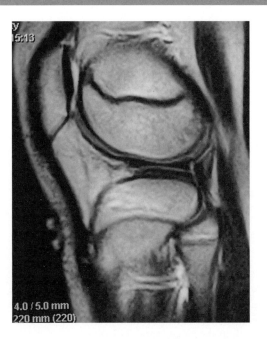

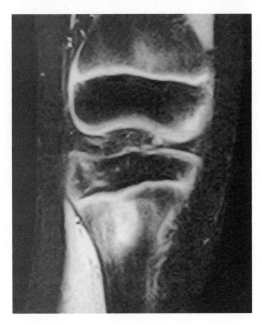

1. What is the diagnosis?
2. What is its cause?
3. What is the essential clinical and radiographic finding of this condition?
4. List some potential complications of this disease.

Osgood-Schlatter Disease

1. Osgood-Schlatter disease.

2. Osteochondrosis of the tibial tuberosity.

3. Soft-tissue swelling in the anterior knee.

4. Nonunion of the bone fragment, patellar subluxation, chondromalacia, avulsion of the patellar tendon, and genu recurvatum.

Reference

Rosenberg ZS, Kawelblum M, Cheung YY, et al: Osgood-Schlatter lesion: Fracture or tendinitis? Scintigraphic, CT, and MR imaging features. Radiology 185:853–858, 1992.

Comments

Osgood-Schlatter disease, an osteochondrosis of the tibial tuberosity, is a disease of adolescents that most commonly affects boys between the ages of 10 and 15 years. Patients present with pain, soft-tissue swelling, and tenderness in the anterior knee in the proximity of the tibial tuberosity. A history of recent athletic activity that includes kicking, jumping, and squatting is typical, and many patients also recall a recent growth spurt. The diagnosis of acute Osgood-Schlatter disease is based on the observations of soft-tissue swelling anterior to the tuberosity and loss of the sharp margination of the patellar tendon. Fragmentation of the tibial tuberosity becomes apparent after 3 to 4 weeks. After the acute stage, a persistent ossific fragment or fragments in a thickened patellar tendon mark the site of previous disease. The diagnosis is made with relative ease using magnetic resonance imaging (MRI). Thickening of the distal patellar tendon, anterior subcutaneous edema, edema in Hoffa's fat pad, and distention of the deep infrapatellar bursa often accompany fragmentation of the tibial tuberosity. Bone marrow edema manifested as areas of low signal intensity on T1W images and high signal intensity on T2W images is occasionally evident in the anterior aspect of the tibial metaphysis and epiphysis.

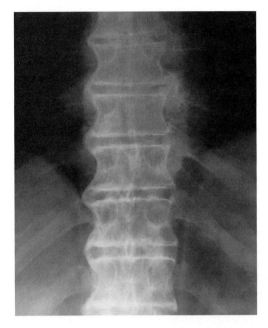 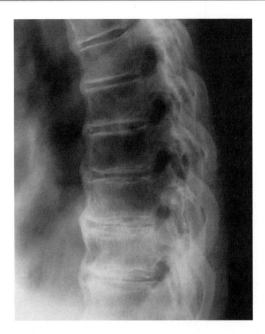

1. Can patients with this disorder present with dysphagia?
2. Why is ossification more pronounced on the right side of the spine?
3. Does ossification progress with aging?
4. List some extraspinal manifestations of this condition.

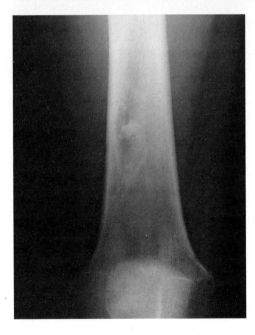 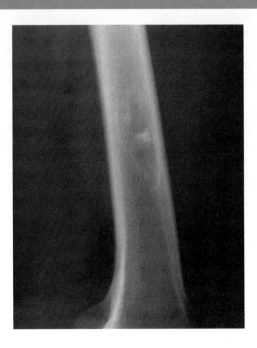

1. How would you describe this lesion?
2. What bone measurement is predictive of the risk for developing pathologic fracture in a tubular bone? What imaging method is most accurate for obtaining this measurement?
3. Bone expansion may be caused by a number of lesions. What tumors can cause expansile metastasis?
4. What imaging features help differentiate a low-grade chondrosarcoma from an enchondroma?

Diffuse Idiopathic Skeletal Hyperostosis

1. Yes, when the cervical spine is involved.

2. The pulsating effect from the thoracic aorta inhibits soft-tissue ossification.

3. Yes, there is an increasing prevalence with aging.

4. Enthesopathy and para-articular bony excrescences.

Reference

Resnick D, Niwayama G: Diffuse idiopathic skeletal hyperostosis (DISH): Ankylosing hyperostosis of Forestier and Rotes-Querol. In Resnick D (ed): Diagnosis of Bone and Joint Disorders. Philadelphia, WB Saunders, pp 1463–1495.

Comments

Diffuse idiopathic skeletal hyperostosis is a disorder common in elderly people and is characterized by undulating soft-tissue calcification and hyperostosis along the anterolateral aspect of the spine involving at least four contiguous vertebral bodies. The clinical manifestations of this condition are generally mild, consisting of restricted motion and tendinitis from enthesopathy. The most common location affected is the thoracic spine. In isolated disease, the intervertebral disks do not undergo degeneration; thus, the disk height is maintained. Laminated calcification and ossification develop along the spine, and the deposited bone may be variable in thickness, ranging from 2 mm to 20 mm. It tends to have a wavy contour protruding at the disk space level, owing to the increased bone deposition at these levels, as well as a more anterior position of the ossification. Radiolucent areas within the ossified mass, also common at the disk level, correspond to disk material that has extended anteriorly. Radiolucent areas between the deposited bone and the vertebral body are characteristically terminated at the superior and inferior margins of the vertebra.

Enthesopathy is a common component of this condition. In the pelvis, ligamentous and tendinous calcification and ossification may occur in the iliac crest, ischium, and trochanteric regions of the femur. Iliolumbar, sacrotuberous, and sacroiliac ligament involvement is typical of diffuse idiopathic skeletal hyperostosis.

Assessment of Bone Lesions

1. Geographic pattern, metadiaphyseal region, sharp margination with a narrow zone of transition, and calcific matrix. No cortical break, periostitis, or soft-tissue mass.

2. Destruction of 50% of the cortical surface. Computed tomography.

3. Renal carcinoma; thyroid carcinoma; hepatoma; and, occasionally, prostate carcinoma, melanoma, and pheochromocytoma.

4. Size exceeding 5 cm, endosteal scalloping, wide zone of transition, periosteal reaction, and presence of pain suggest a chondrosarcoma.

Reference

Manaster BJ: Tumors. In Handbook of Skeletal Radiology, 2nd ed. St. Louis, Mosby, 1997, pp 1–4.

Comments

When evaluating a bone lesion, you should always know the patient's age, the patient's sex, and whether there are constitutional signs of an underlying disease process. Then you should make several important observations before embarking on a differential diagnostic list. Is the pattern of bone destruction geographic, moth-eaten, or permeative? Is the lesion located in the diaphysis, metaphysis, or epiphysis? Is the zone of transition sharp or poorly marginated? Is the margin sclerotic or nonsclerotic? Does it have any tumor matrix, and, if so, is it chondroid or osteoid? Is the cortex disrupted or scalloped, or is there periostitis? Is there an associated soft-tissue mass? This lesion shows characteristic features of a benign tumor (i.e., small size, narrow zone of transition with sclerotic margin, no endosteal scalloping or periostitis, and no soft-tissue mass).

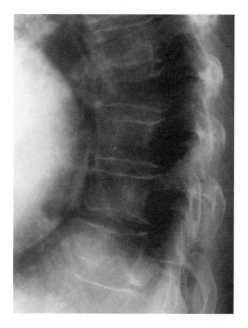 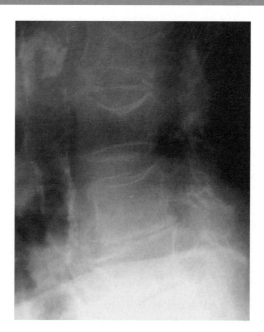

1. What do you observe, and what conditions would you include in your differential diagnosis?
2. In the appendicular skeleton, what radiographic sign indicates rapid bone loss?
3. What is the preferred imaging technique for diagnosing diminished bone density?
4. How much heparin must be administered to induce osteoporosis? Is it permanent?

Osteoporosis

1. Osteopenia and biconcave vertebral bodies. Senile osteoporosis, medication, endocrine disorders, nutritional deficiency states, alcoholism, marrow replacement processes, liver disease, anemia, and osteogenesis imperfecta.

2. Cortical tunneling.

3. Dual photon absorptiometry.

4. More than 15,000 units per day. No.

Reference

Raymakers JA, Kapelle JW, van Beresteijn EC, Duursma SA: Assessment of osteoporotic spine deformity. A new method. Skeletal Radiol 19:91–97, 1990.

Comments

Osteoporosis refers to a generalized decrease in bone mass caused by a deficiency of osteoid formation or by increased bone resorption. It can involve the entire skeleton (generalized), one segment of the skeleton (regional), or one or more focal areas (localized). Generalized osteoporosis can be caused by numerous conditions. The radiographic manifestations caused by many of these processes predominate in the axial skeleton and produce changes relatively early in the spine. Resorption of the horizontal trabeculae in the vertebral body causes a loss of bone density while increasing the conspicuity of the vertical trabeculation. Cortical thinning also occurs, but the end plates remain prominent. Changes in the vertebral body contour can occur from compression fractures and protrusion of the intervertebral disks. Generalized height loss and a characteristic biconcave deformity (as seen in this patient) are common findings in senile and postmenopausal osteoporosis. Anterior wedging and diffuse compression fractures are also common manifestations and can contribute to significant kyphosis in the thoracic spine. Bone pain can be associated with an acute loss of height of a vertebral body, but it is often difficult, even with comparison radiographs, to determine the age of a vertebral body deformity.

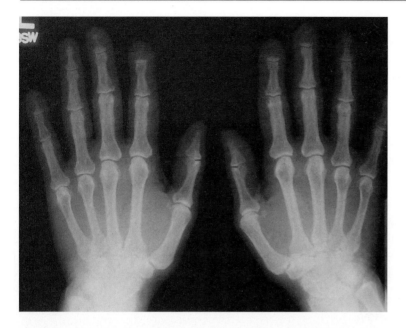

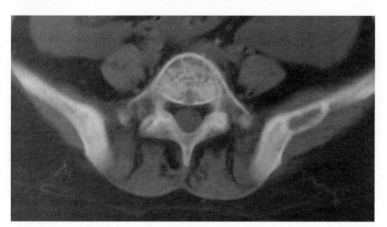

1. Do you think this patient's serum calcium level is elevated?
2. What are the primary causes of this disease and their relative incidence?
3. What is the radiologic hallmark of this disease?
4. What would you consider a good screening radiographic series for this disorder?

Hyperparathyroidism

1. Only if the patient has the primary form of hyper-parathyroidism.

2. Single parathyroid adenoma (50%–80%), multiple adenomas (10%), parathyroid hyperplasia (10%–40%), and carcinoma (rare).

3. Bone resorption.

4. Radiographs of the hand, pelvis, and shoulders.

Reference

Pugh DG: Subperiosteal resorption of bone. A roentgenologic manifestation of primary hyperparathyroidism and renal osteodystrophy. AJR Am J Roentgenol 66:577–586, 1951.

Comments

Hyperparathyroidism refers to a group of disorders characterized by the presence of increased circulating parathyroid hormone (PTH). The presence of excess PTH results in increased osteoclastic resorption of the bone. Osteocytic osteolysis is responsible for the initial calcium release from the bone. In primary hyperparathyroidism, the parathyroid gland overproduces PTH. Patients present with weakness, lethargy, bone pain, polydipsia, and polyuria. Other associated abnormalities include nephrolithiasis, gastrointestinal ulcers, and pancreatitis. Common causes of the primary form of the disease include adenoma, hyperplasia of the gland, parathyroid carcinoma, tumors that secrete PTH-like substances, and type 2 multiple endocrine neoplasia. Secondary hyperparathyroidism occurs in response to chronic hypocalcemia, usually from renal glomerular disease and sometimes from malabsorption. *Tertiary hyperparathyroidism* refers to an autonomous gland that has escaped the regulatory effects of serum calcium after a prolonged period of stimulation; this typically occurs in patients who are on chronic hemodialysis.

Bone resorption (particularly subperiosteal) is the radiologic hallmark of hyperparathyroidism. This patient, who has secondary hyperparathyroidism from chronic renal failure induced by diabetes mellitus, demonstrates classic findings of acro-osteolysis and subperiosteal resorption of the cortices on the radial surface of the middle phalanges. Other common preferred sites of bone resorption are the distal clavicle; the medial metaphyseal surfaces of the proximal femur, humerus, and tibia; the distal metaphysis of the radius and ulna; the symphysis pubis; and the sacroiliac joints. A brown tumor is evident in the left ilium.

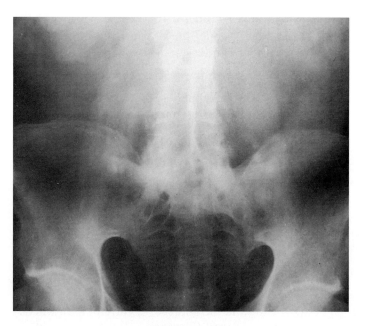
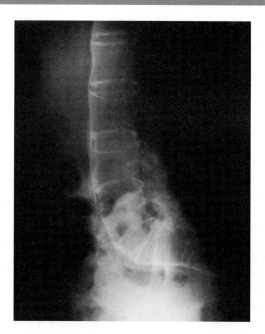

1. What are the radiographic findings?
2. What is the incidence of positive human leukocyte antigen B27 (HLA-B27) in the general population?
3. List some extra-articular manifestations of this disease.
4. List some complications that can occur in this patient's spine.

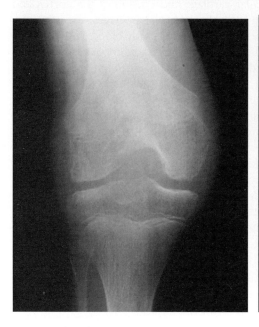
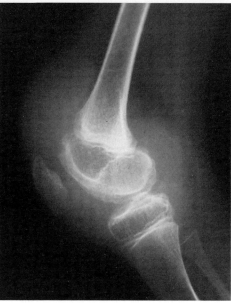

1. List the differential diagnosis.
2. In the frontal view of the knee, what caused widening of the intercondylar notch?
3. In patients with this disease, what is meant by a pseudotumor? Where are pseudotumors common?
4. What is one sequela of hemorrhage into the epiphyseal cartilage (growth plate)?

CASE 10

Ankylosing Spondylitis

1. Syndesmophytes ("bamboo spine"), interspinous ligament ossification, and ankylosis of the sacroiliac joints.

2. Six to eight percent of the population are positive.

3. Iritis, aortic insufficiency, and interstitial lung disease.

4. Pseudoarthrosis, fractures, atlantoaxial instability, spondylodiscitis, cord compression, and spinal stenosis.

Reference

Van der Linden S, van der Heijde D: Ankylosing spondylitis. Clinical features. Rheum Dis Clin North Am 24:663–676, 1998.

Comments

This case is an "aunt Minnie." The unmistakable features of ankylosing spondylitis (AS) are evident in both radiographs. AS is the most common seronegative spondyloarthropathy and has an overwhelmingly male predilection. The onset of the disease occurs between ages 15 and 35 years, and more than 90% of those afflicted are HLA-B27 positive. Clinically, these patients present with low back pain and stiffness. The sacroiliac joint is classically the first site involved, and sacroiliitis is a hallmark of the disease. Initial periarticular osteoporosis and superficial cortical erosions on the iliac side of the joint are followed by more dramatic erosive changes that result in joint space widening. Eburnation develops as a dense, ill-defined band of sclerosis. As proliferative changes become more prominent, irregular bony bridges eventually lead to complete joint ankylosis. All these findings occur in both the ligamentous and the synovial portions of the joint.

Bamboo spine is a term that characterizes the presence of extensive formation of syndesmophytes (ossification of the annulus fibrosis). The "trolley track" sign is seen in frontal radiographs and denotes three vertically oriented, dense lines corresponding to ossification of the supraspinous and interspinous ligaments and apophyseal joint capsules. The trolley track sign may be preceded by the "dagger" sign, which is a single radiodense line on frontal radiographs indicating ossification of the supraspinous and interspinous ligaments.

CASE 11

Hemophiliac Arthropathy

1. Hemophilia, septic arthritis, and, sometimes, juvenile rheumatoid arthritis.

2. Hemorrhage into the cruciate ligament attachments.

3. Intraosseous or subperiosteal hemorrhage giving the appearance of an expansile lytic process. Ilium, femur, and tibia.

4. Growth discrepancy.

Reference

Kulkarni MV, Drolshagen LF, Kaye JJ, et al: MR imaging of hemophiliac arthropathy. J Comput Assist Tomogr 10:445–449, 1986.

Comments

Hemophilia is an X-linked genetic disorder caused by a deficiency of coagulation factor VIII, resulting in a coagulopathy. In hemophilia, recurrent intra-articular hemorrhages occur frequently. The knee and elbow are particularly vulnerable to repeated injuries. When repeated intra-articular hemorrhages occur, the irritating effect of the blood within the joint causes the development of a chronic synovitis. Increased blood flow from chronic synovitis is responsible for periarticular osteopenia and accelerated bone growth. The hypertrophied synovial membrane (pannus) causes degeneration of the articular cartilage and erosion of the cortex and subchondral bone. In acute hemorrhages, the joint capsule may become distended with blood and diminish the range of motion. This effusion appears more radiodense than do nonhemorrhagic effusions; this is a useful observation for narrowing the differential possibilities. Always remember that an acute hemorrhage may mimic a septic joint. Soft-tissue swelling and warmth about the joint are common findings, and fever, increased erythrocyte sedimentation rate, and elevation of white blood cell levels may be present. In chronic cases, the deposition of hemosiderin in the tissues may lead to areas of increased density in the joint that mimic calcification on radiographs but are unequivocal on magnetic resonance imaging.

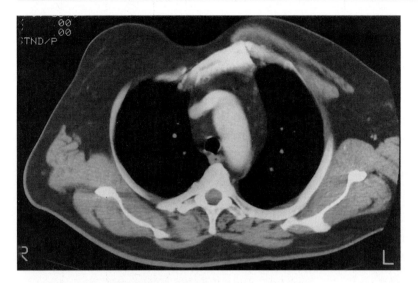

1. What is the principal finding?

2. What diagnosis does this finding bring to mind? What appendicular abnormality is associated with this finding?

3. What is syndactyly, and what are its types?

4. What is the differential diagnosis for syndactyly?

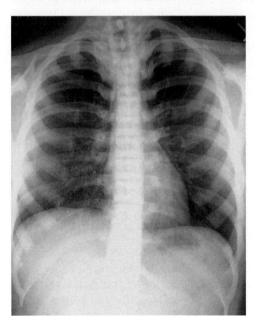 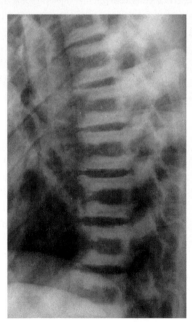 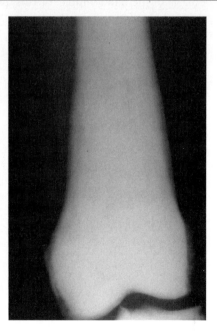

1. What is this disease? List some cranial abnormalities.

2. What common complication occurs in the mandible?

3. What is the differential for dense metaphyseal bands?

4. Engelmann's disease also causes generalized increased bone density in children. How does the appearance of this disease differ from osteopetrosis?

C A S E 1 2

Poland's Syndrome

1. Unilateral absence of the pectoralis muscles.

2. Poland's syndrome. Syndactyly.

3. A lack of differentiation between two or more digits. Can be either fibrous or osseous and either partial or complete.

4. Apert's syndrome, Ellis-van Creveld syndrome, acrocephalopolysyndactyly, chondrodysplasia punctata, Down's syndrome, Fanconi's syndrome, Laurence-Moon-Biedl syndrome, neurofibromatosis, Pierre Robin syndrome, thrombocytopenia–absent radius syndrome, and trisomy 13 and 18 syndromes.

Reference

Swischuk LE, Stansberry SD: Radiographic manifestations of anomalies of the chest wall. Radiol Clin North Am 29:271-277, 1991.

Comments

This "aunt Minnie" is characterized by unilateral absence of the pectoral muscles and ipsilateral syndactyly. The chest wall deformity may be either a partial or a complete absence of the greater pectoral muscle. Additional anomalies included in this syndrome are hypoplasia of the hand, nipple, or ribs; pectus excavatum; pectus carinatum; elevated scapulae; carpal coalition; tendon abnormalities; and scoliosis. There also is an association with dextrocardia.

C A S E 1 3

Osteopetrosis

1. Osteopetrosis. Hydrocephalus, optic nerve atrophy, facial paralysis, deafness, subarachnoid hemorrhage, and obliteration of the sinuses.

2. Osteomyelitis.

3. Heavy metal poisoning, hypothyroidism, scurvy, congenital syphilis, healed rickets, and systemic illness.

4. Engelmann's disease affects only the diaphysis of a tubular bone, whereas osteopetrosis involves the entire bone. Engelmann's disease rarely affects the bones of the hands and feet, clavicles, pelvis, ribs, and scapula.

Reference

Greenspan A: Sclerosing bone dysplasias—a target-site approach. Skeletal Radiol 20:561-583, 1991.

Comments

Osteopetrosis, or Albers-Schönberg disease, is a rare hereditary bone disease caused by lack of absorption of the primary spongiosa in the process of enchondral bone formation. It is suspected that an underlying enzyme deficiency is responsible for this lack of absorption because the vascular mesenchyme that erodes the spongiosa fails to form. Clinically, the disease varies in its severity and age of presentation. Two forms of osteopetrosis are recognized. A congenital form is inherited as an autosomal recessive trait and is lethal. Hepatosplenomegaly and anemia are characteristics of this form, and the infant, if not stillborn at birth, fails to thrive. The tarda form is inherited as an autosomal dominant trait and is clinically benign, although pathologic fractures are a prominent feature of the disease. Organomegaly and anemia do not occur. Poor dentition may lead to osteomyelitis of the maxilla and mandible. The key to this case is that the bones are too dense. Radiographically, osteopetrosis is characterized by a symmetrical, generalized increase in bone density with loss of distinction between the cortical and the medullary bones. Failure of tubulation results in an "Erlenmeyer flask" deformity. A "bone-in-bone" appearance may be evident in the long bones and spine. Other findings in the spine include diffuse vertebral body sclerosis or increased density only at the end plates (sandwich vertebrae sign). The increased density in the skull affects both the base and the calvaria, obliterating the diploic space.

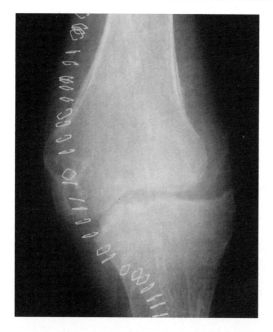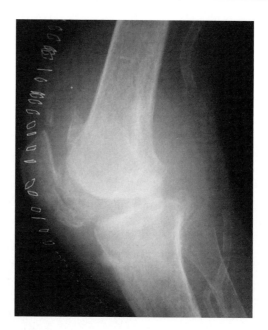

1. By what mechanisms could the joint have become this way?
2. Identify the potential sequelae of this process.
3. Early in the disease process, what else might you consider in the differential diagnosis?
4. What peculiar manifestations of hematogenous osteomyelitis do intravenous drug abusers demonstrate?

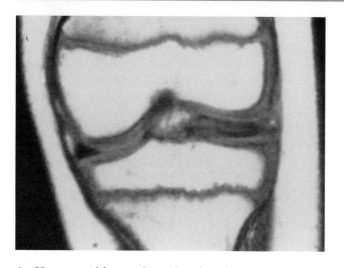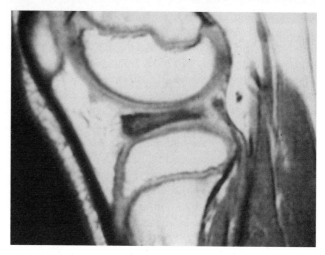

1. How would you describe the abnormality?
2. What is the leading hypothesis for the development of this congenital variant? Which side is more common, lateral or medial meniscus?
3. What will eventually happen to this meniscus, and when?
4. How do these patients present?

Septic Arthritis

1. Hematogenous spread, direct extension, or direct implantation of bacteria into the joint.

2. Osteonecrosis, degenerative joint disease, and occasionally, bony ankylosis. Sepsis is also a very real concern.

3. Anything that causes synovial inflammation such as crystal deposition diseases (hydroxyapatite disease, gout, pseudogout), hemophilia, juvenile chronic arthritis, and neuroarthropathy.

4. Unusual locations (spine, sacroiliac joints) and unusual organisms (*Pseudomonas, Klebsiella, Serratia*).

References

Ma LD, Frassica FJ, Bluemke DA, Fishman EK: CT and MRI evaluation of musculoskeletal infection. Crit Rev Diagn Imaging 38:535–568, 1997.

Perry CR: Septic arthritis. Am J Orthop 28:168–178, 1999.

Comments

Infection of a joint is a serious problem. It is a condition that should be diagnosed rapidly, particularly in immunocompromised patients. This patient demonstrates classic signs of advanced disease. *Staphylococcus* and *Gonococcus* are the infectious agents responsible for a majority of cases of septic arthropathy. Clinically, patients complain of pain, erythema, soft-tissue swelling, and effusion. Patients may present with leukocytosis and fever. You should always consider this diagnosis when inflammation is observed that involves only one joint. The initial findings are related to synovial inflammation (focal periarticular osteopenia), but osseous destruction can be rapid once a pannus has formed. The joint becomes irregularly narrowed as the pannus penetrates through the cartilage or into the recesses of the joint, producing central and marginal erosions. As cartilage destruction progresses, the joint narrowing becomes widespread. Periostitis in the periarticular region of the infected bone is a common finding, although it is often subtle. The most important test that should be performed in patients suspected of having an infected joint is aspiration. Although this procedure may not always identify the bacterial agent, it will demonstrate the presence of leukocytes, an elevated protein count, and a low sugar level, which are diagnostic of septic arthropathy. Infections in the foot and the hand should be further evaluated with magnetic resonance imaging, because it gives a better anatomic delineation of the extent of infection.

Discoid Lateral Meniscus

1. Degenerated discoid lateral meniscus.

2. Abnormal inferior fascicular attachment of the posterior horn contributes to discoid growth. Lateral.

3. A discoid meniscus degenerates early because weight-bearing forces are not distributed properly. A majority of cases will tear by early adulthood.

4. Clicking, pain, effusion, and locking are common clinical symptoms in childhood.

References

Ryu KN, Kim IS, Ahn JW, et al: MR imaging of tears of discoid lateral menisci. AJR Am J Roentgenol 171:963–967, 1998.

Silverman JM, Mink JH, Deutsch AL: Discoid menisci of the knee: MR imaging appearance. Radiology 173:351–354, 1989.

Comments

A discoid meniscus is a morphologic variant characterized by poor constriction of the central portion of the meniscus and thickening of its free end. Most experts believe that it represents a developmental defect resulting from abnormal peripheral attachments. Owing to the thickened morphology, there is an abnormal extension of fibrocartilage between the femoral condyle and the tibial plateau that is more susceptible to trauma. The aim of treatment is resection of this unstable free-end segment. Clinically, patients present with symptoms of a meniscal tear. Lateral discoid meniscus has been classified into six types. Type 1 represents a thick, rounded slab with parallel superior and inferior surfaces. Type 2 represents a biconcave type with a thin central portion similar to the configuration of a red blood cell. Type 3 is a wedge type that is generally smaller than type 1 discoid meniscus. Type 4 is asymmetrical, with an anterior horn larger than the posterior horn. Type 5 represents a variation of type 1 but is less severe. Type 6 represents any of the first five types, but with extensive tears. The diagnosis can be made easily on magnetic resonance imaging by the absence of the normal triangular meniscal morphology. You should suspect a discoid meniscus when a "bow tie" is present on three or more consecutive sagittal sections.

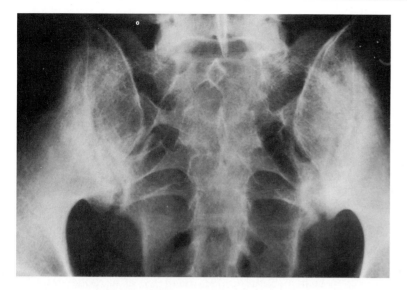

1. Predominant involvement of the ilium in patients with sacroiliitis is theorized to be related to what?
2. What inflammatory bowel diseases are classically associated with sacroiliitis? Are there any others?
3. Eventually, who is more likely to get sacroiliac joint ankylosis—a patient with enteropathic sacroiliitis, psoriasis, or Reiter's syndrome?
4. How is a Ferguson view performed?

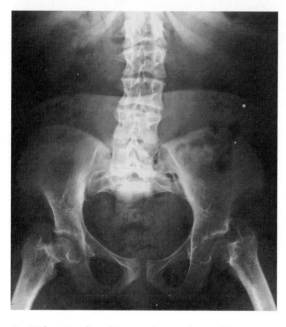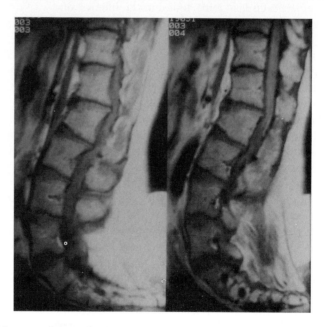

1. What is the diagnosis, and would you consider anything else?
2. What is a "trident hand," and when is this deformity typically seen?
3. Genetically, what is the risk for developing the homozygous form of this disease?
4. What are some characteristic findings in the skull? What can be a complication of this morphology?

Sacroiliitis

1. The ilium has thinner cartilage than the sacrum has and also possesses degenerative clefts and perpendicular splits in the cartilage.

2. Ulcerative colitis and Crohn's disease. Whipple's disease, infectious colitis with *Salmonella, Shigella,* and *Yersinia,* and intestinal bypass surgery.

3. Enteropathic sacroiliitis.

4. Anteroposterior radiograph of the pelvis with the tube angulated 25 to 30 degrees in a cephalad direction.

References

Battistone MJ, Manaster BJ, Reda DJ, Clegg DO: Radiographic diagnosis of sacroiliitis—are sacroiliac views really better? J Rheumatol 25:2395-2401, 1998.

Oostveen J, Prevo R, den Boer J, van de Laar M: Early detection of sacroiliitis on magnetic resonance imaging and subsequent development of sacroiliitis on plain radiography. A prospective, longitudinal study. J Rheumatol 26:1953-1958, 1999.

Comments

The principal observation when evaluating sacroiliitis is the distribution of the disease. Typically, the synovial portion of the sacroiliac joint, found in the inferior one half to two thirds of the joint on frontal radiographs, is more severely involved than is the ligamentous portion. Erosions involving the synovial articulation affect the iliac side greater than the sacral articulation. In ankylosing spondylitis, the disease is generally bilateral and symmetrical in distribution. Sacroiliitis associated with inflammatory bowel disease is usually bilateral and symmetrical in distribution and cannot be differentiated from ankylosing spondylitis. Psoriatic arthropathy and Reiter's syndrome result in osseous erosions and bony sclerosis that are similar to those seen in ankylosing spondylitis, although ankylosis is less common. The distribution may be bilateral and symmetrical, bilateral and asymmetrical, or unilateral. Osteoarthritis may involve one or both joints and is manifested by joint space narrowing, osteophyte formation, and eburnation. When only one sacroiliac joint appears abnormal, one must always consider the possibility of infection, particularly if there is a history of intravenous drug use. In this situation, it is best to aspirate the joint, although magnetic resonance imaging and computed tomography may be noninvasive alternatives. Both cross-sectional imaging techniques allow direct inspection of the joint surface and are better able to detect cartilaginous and osseous destruction than is conventional radiography.

Achondroplasia

1. Achondroplasia. Usually the findings are distinctive, although milder forms of this dwarfism such as hypochondroplasia and chondrohypoplasia (spares the skull) and chondrodystrophia calcificans congenita (affects only one side) may occasionally be considered.

2. Divergence of the middle and ring fingers occurring in infants with achondroplasia.

3. The same likelihood as that of having normal offspring—25%.

4. Large skull, frontal bossing, short skull base, anteriorly displaced foramen magnum. Hydrocephalus.

Reference

Lemyre E, Azouz EM, Teebi AS, et al: Bone dysplasia series. Achondroplasia, hypochondroplasia and thanatophoric dysplasia: Review and update. Can Assoc Radiol J 50:185-197, 1999.

Comments

Achondroplasia is a bone dysplasia characterized by rhizomelic, short-limbed dwarfism. Eighty to ninety percent of cases occur as a sporadic mutation, and the remaining cases are inherited as an autosomal dominant trait. The essential abnormality is a defect in enchondral bone formation affecting all bones formed in cartilage. It is the most common form of dwarfism, and bone deformities are evident at birth. In the tubular bones, ossification of the periosteum exceeds cartilaginous ossification, causing the new bone to extend beyond the margins of the growth plate. The bone appears short and square with cupped ends. In the spine, the spinal canal is narrowed in both transverse and anteroposterior dimensions. Progressive narrowing of the interpediculate distance and shortening of the pedicles contribute to significant spinal stenosis. The vertebral bodies are also shortened in the anteroposterior dimension and show prominent posterior scalloping. The lumbosacral lordosis is exaggerated, resulting in a horizontal sacrum. In some patients, a progressive gibbus deformity at the thoracolumbar spine may compress the spinal cord. Classic findings are evident in the pelvis, where there is shortening of the iliac bones and narrowing of the sacrum. The morphologic changes in the innominate bones result in small, deep, greater sciatic notches, squaring of the iliac wings, and flattening of the acetabular angles ("champagne glass" appearance).

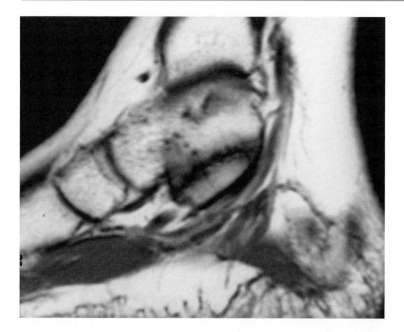

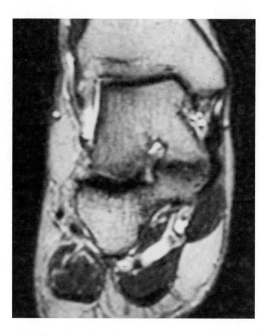

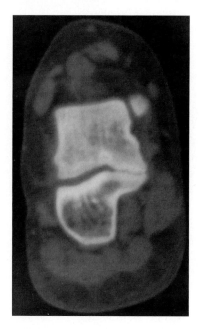

1. What is the diagnosis? How often is this process bilateral?
2. What is the essential embryologic abnormality?
3. What is the preferred imaging technique for diagnosis and preoperative planning?
4. What are some radiographic findings of a calcaneonavicular coalition?

Talocalcaneal Tarsal Coalition

1. Talocalcaneal fibrous coalition. 20% to 25%.

2. Failure of tarsal bone segmentation.

3. Computed tomography (CT) or magnetic resonance imaging (MRI), although MRI allows for more flexibility in the imaging planes and is superior for establishing other causes of ankle pain.

4. Loss of normal space between the calcaneus and the tarsal navicular, hypoplasia of the head of the talus, and elongation of the anterior calcaneal process.

Reference

Emery KH, Bisset GS 3rd, Johnson ND, Nunan PJ: Tarsal coalition: A blinded comparison of MRI and CT. Pediatr Radiol 28:612-616, 1998.

Comments

This case is as straightforward as they come. A talocalcaneal coalition is one of the most common types of tarsal coalition, along with a calcaneonavicular coalition. Other tarsal coalitions include calcaneocuboid and talonavicular coalitions. Talocalcaneal coalitions usually elicit pain and diminished range of motion. Coalitions often occur in both feet, and, occasionally, more than one type of coalition may be seen in one foot. There are three types of coalitions. An osseous coalition is characterized by the presence of a bony bar that extends between two tarsal bones. Generally, if complete fusion occurs, it does so by the 12th year of life. Eburnation or sclerosis and close approximation between the osseous surfaces of two bones characterize fibrous and cartilaginous coalitions, the two other types of coalitions. Almost all talocalcaneal fusions occur in the middle facet. Radiographically, the diagnosis may be established if one identifies a talar beak, broadening of the lateral talar process, narrowing of the posterior subtalar joint, concave undersurface of the talar neck, failure to visualize the middle subtalar joint, and a ball-and-socket ankle joint. Both CT and MRI are very good for detecting tarsal coalitions and are advocated for preoperative evaluation. In this case, a fibrous coalition was confirmed at surgery.

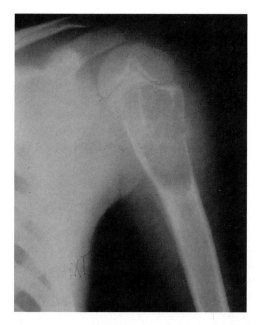

1. Describe the "fallen fragment" sign. Where is it most commonly seen?
2. What is meant by a "pseudotrabeculated" radiographic appearance?
3. At what age do most pathologic fractures that are related to this lesion occur?
4. When does this lesion stop growing?

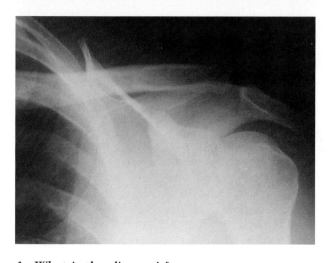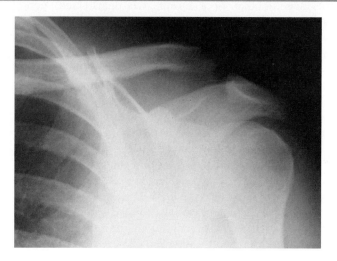

1. What is the diagnosis?
2. List some complications of this injury.
3. What two steps are critical in diagnosing a type 2 separation? What is considered a significant finding?
4. What is a "floating clavicle"?

Simple Bone Cyst

1. Detached fragment of bone in the dependent portion of a cyst cavity. A simple bone cyst in the humerus.

2. Ridges between areas of endosteal scalloping give the appearance of coarsened trabeculation. There is no osseous matrix in the cyst itself.

3. The highest incidence occurs at about 10 years of age.

4. With epiphyseal closure.

References

Chigira M, Maehara S, Arita S, Udagawa E: The aetiology and treatment of simple bone cysts. J Bone Joint Surg Br 65:633–637, 1983.

Makley JT, Joyce MJ: Unicameral bone cyst (simple bone cyst). Orthop Clin North Am 20:407–415, 1989.

Comments

A simple, or unicameral, bone cyst is common, and this lesion is a true fluid-filled cavity with a wall of fibrous tissue. Most of these cysts are discovered in people younger than 20 years. Males are twice as likely as females to have them. In adults, simple cysts have a predilection for the calcaneus and the innominate bones of the pelvis. In children and adolescents, 90% to 95% of cysts involve the long bones. The radiographic appearance is that of a lucent, well-demarcated, geographic lesion that has its long axis parallel to the axis of the bone. It arises in the metaphysis but may migrate into the diaphysis with skeletal growth. The cyst is broader toward the metaphysis than it is toward the diaphysis. Abnormal remodeling of the bone is noticeable, and the cortex occasionally appears expanded. A rim of sclerosis surrounding the lesion is variable in thickness but may be absent. Cortical disruption and periosteal reaction do not occur unless there is a pathologic fracture through the lesion. On magnetic resonance imaging, the typical features of a simple cyst are low signal intensity on T1W images and uniformly increased signal intensity on T2W images. Remember that hemorrhage in the cyst may alter its magnetic resonance imaging appearance.

Acromioclavicular Joint Dislocations

1. Type 3 acromioclavicular (AC) joint dislocation.

2. Heterotopic calcification-ossification, posttraumatic osteolysis of the distal clavicle, and secondary osteoarthritis.

3. Stress (weight-bearing) views and comparison with the contralateral shoulder. A difference of 3 to 4 mm when compared with the normal shoulder, or a change in alignment with weight bearing.

4. Simultaneous dislocation of the AC and sternoclavicular joints.

Reference

Rockwood CA Jr: Subluxations and dislocations about the shoulder. Injuries to the acromioclavicular joint. In Rockwood CA, Green DP (eds): Fracture in Adults, 2nd ed. Philadelphia, JB Lippincott, 1984, pp 860–910.

Comments

AC joint separations-dislocations occur from direct impaction to the point of the shoulder. The most widely used classification is the Allman classification, which identifies three different types. The radiographs appear normal in a type 1 separation. On magnetic resonance imaging, soft-tissue swelling about the joint and effusion may be evident and indicate a mild strain of the AC and coracoclavicular ligaments. In a type 2 injury, there is disruption of the AC ligament and partial disruption of the coracoclavicular ligaments, such that the clavicle migrates superiorly less than 5 mm or 50% of the width of the clavicle on weight-bearing views. In type 3 injuries, the AC and coracoclavicular ligaments are completely disrupted, and there is clavicular migration exceeding 5 mm or 50% of the bone width. Disruption of the coracoclavicular ligaments is a conspicuous finding on T2W coronal and sagittal images of the shoulder. Fiber disruption and edema or hemorrhage are common magnetic resonance imaging features at the site of ligament failure. Rockwood described three additional injury patterns. In type 4 injuries, the clavicle is displaced posteriorly into or through the trapezius muscle. In type 5 injuries, the clavicle migrates superiorly more than in a type 3 separation. In type 6 injuries, the clavicle dislocates inferiorly below the coracoid or acromion process.

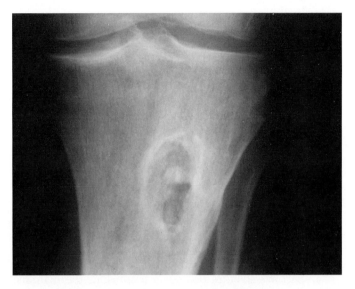

1. List the entities that you would consider.
2. Describe Garré's sclerosing osteitis.
3. What percentage of patients with Brodie's abscess have a sequestrum?
4. If this lesion is identified in a child, what should you look for?

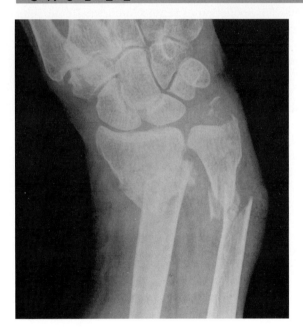

1. Describe the Frykman classification.
2. What are the goals for reduction of a distal radius fracture?
3. What is Smith's fracture?
4. How does Barton's fracture differ from Smith's fracture?

Brodie's Abscess

1. Brodie's abscess; fibrous dysplasia; occasionally, simple bone cyst.

2. Uncommon manifestation of a low-grade infection, which causes a sclerotic reaction without bone destruction or sequestration.

3. About 20%.

4. Communication to the growth plate by a tortuous sinus tract.

Reference

Lopes TD, Reinus WR, Wilson AJ: Quantitative analysis of the plain radiographic appearance of Brodie's abscess. Invest Radiol 32:51–58, 1997.

Comments

When a bone infection becomes a chronic condition, it may produce a spectrum of radiographic appearances. Brodie's abscess is a painful lesion characterized by a well-defined geographic, radiolucent focus surrounded by diffuse sclerosis. Two thirds of these lesions occur in the metaphysis of a bone, whereas the remaining one third of lesions occur in the diaphysis. Brodie's abscess represents a cavity in the bone lined by inflammatory granulation tissue and is filled with purulent or mucoid fluid. It is hypothesized that the bone abscess develops when the organism has a reduced virulence or when the host demonstrates increased resistance to the infection. Several findings suggested the correct diagnosis in this case. The location and appearance of the lesion are nonspecific, but did you notice the involucrum in the lateral tibial cortex and the sequestrum?

Distal Radius Fracture

1. The Frykman classification consists of eight types that describe Colles' fractures. Type 1 is extra-articular. Type 3 is intra-articular to the radiocarpal joint. Type 5 is intra-articular to the distal radioulnar joint. Type 7 is intra-articular to both the radiocarpal joint and the distal radioulnar joint. Types 2, 4, 6, and 8 denote the presence of a concomitant ulnar styloid fracture to the preceding type.

2. Maintenance of radial length, 0- to 10-degree palmar tilt, 14-degree ulnar inclination, and articular congruity.

3. Fracture of the distal radial metaphysis or epiphysis, with or without articular involvement, which displaces or angulates volarly.

4. Barton's fracture denotes a fracture of the marginal rim of the radius that displaces along with the carpus, in essence representing a fracture-subluxation. Therefore, a volar Barton's fracture appears identical to a Thomas type 2 Smith's fracture.

References

Jupiter JB: Fractures of the distal end of the radius. J Bone Joint Surg Am 73:461–469, 1991.

Thomas FB: Reduction of Smith's fractures. J Bone Joint Surg Br 39:463–470, 1957.

Comments

Fractures of the distal radius are very common. In this case, the lateral view is withheld so that we may discuss different types of fractures. In the adult, the most common fracture is Colles' fracture (distal radial metaphysis or epiphysis fracture with dorsal cortical comminution). The mechanism of injury is usually a fall on an outstretched hand. There are numerous classifications for Colles' fractures, but the Frykman classification is useful for prognosis. On the basis of the radiograph, this would be a Frykman type 6 Colles' fracture, because the fracture extends to the distal radioulnar joint and the ulnar styloid is involved. Smith's fractures are similar except that they displace or angulate in the volar direction; hence, they are frequently referred to as *reverse Colles' fractures*. The Thomas classification describes three types. Type 1 is transverse extra-articular, type 2 is volar intra-articular, and type 3 is oblique juxta-articular. If this patient had Smith's fracture, it would be a type 1 fracture. Most experts prefer to call a type 2 Smith's fracture a volar-type Barton's fracture.

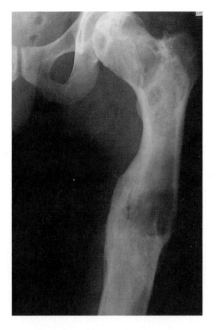 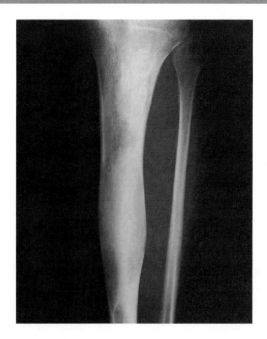

1. What is the diagnosis?
2. Describe McCune-Albright syndrome. How frequently is it seen, and in whom?
3. Can this condition undergo malignant transformation? If so, into what?
4. What is cherubism?

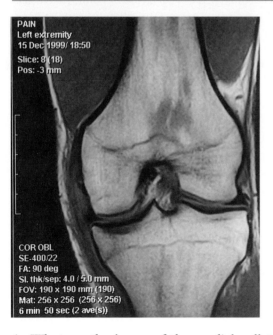 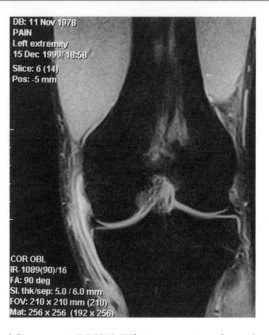

1. What are the layers of the medial collateral ligament (MCL)? What separates these layers?
2. Describe the course of the MCL.
3. How do most injuries to the MCL occur? What part of the MCL is affected?
4. What is a Pellegrini-Stieda lesion? Describe its radiographic appearance.

C A S E 2 3

Fibrous Dysplasia

1. Fibrous dysplasia.

2. Endocrine dysfunction (particularly precocious puberty), café-au-lait pigmentation, and fibrous dysplasia. Thirty percent of females with polyostotic disease.

3. Yes, in less than 1% of cases. Osteosarcoma, fibrosarcoma, and chondrosarcoma. One third of these patients have a previous history of radiation therapy.

4. Familial fibrous dysplasia characterized by bilateral expansile lesions in the mandible associated with multilocular cystic areas.

Reference

Tehranzadeh J, Fung Y, Donohue M, et al: Computed tomography of Paget disease of the skull versus fibrous dysplasia. Skeletal Radiol 27:664–672, 1998.

Comments

Fibrous dysplasia is a disorder caused by a defect in the germ plasm involving the proliferation and maturation of fibroblasts. The marrow becomes replaced by fibrous tissue. The variable amount of osteoid accounts for a wide range of radiographic densities in the bone. Clinically, patients are young and generally present in the first or second decades of life with pain or pathologic fractures. Note that this patient has had fractures of both the femur and the distal tibia. Patients with polyostotic disease frequently have café-au-lait spots (30%–50%), but skin pigmentation is not prominent in the monostotic form of the disease.

Fibrous dysplasia may occur in any bone. The monostotic form has an affinity for the long bones and has a wide spectrum of radiographic appearances, ranging from fairly dense to relatively lytic. When a characteristic, uniform, ground-glass appearance (as in this case) is seen centrally within the medullary cavity, the diagnosis is straightforward. The endosteal surface may be scalloped. Expansion of the bone is common, as are bowing deformities. Lesions that have been present for a long period of time may demonstrate spotty calcification or a well-defined sclerotic rim. Pathologic fractures, owing to weakening of the bone, can elicit a periosteal reaction, but otherwise periostitis is not a typical feature of this condition.

C A S E 2 4

Medial Collateral Ligament Tear

1. There are two layers: the tibiocollateral ligament (superficial layer) and the meniscofemoral and meniscotibial ligaments (deep layer). A small bursa.

2. Arises from the epicondylar portion of the medial femoral condyle and attaches to the medial tibia about 5 cm below the joint line.

3. Valgus injury to a flexed knee. Proximal anterior fibers.

4. Posttraumatic calcification-ossification of the proximal attachment of the MCL. Arcuate, radiodense collection of calcification or ossification arising from the epicondylar portion of the medial femoral condyle.

References

Rasenberg EI, Lemmens JA, van Kampen A, et al: Grading medial collateral ligament injury: Comparison of MR imaging and instrumented valgus-varus laxity test-device. A prospective double-blind study. Eur J Radiol 21:18–24, 1995.

Schweitzer ME, Tran D, Deely DM, Hume EL: Medial collateral ligament injuries: Evaluation of multiple signs, prevalence and location of associated bone bruises, and assessment with MR imaging. Radiology 194:825–829, 1995.

Comments

The MCL is composed of two layers of connective tissue separated by a small bursa. The fibers of the MCL are taut when the knee is extended and help prevent hyperextension. The MCL remains taut throughout flexion, helping prevent valgus angulation when the knee is flexed. Most injuries occur when the knee is flexed and a valgus stress is applied to the knee.

Injuries to the MCL may be graded according to its magnetic resonance imaging (MRI) appearance, although some reports question the accuracy of MRI for classification of MCL injuries. A grade 1 strain is characterized by perifascicular edema paralleling the tibiocollateral ligament but with preservation of its morphology. In grade 2 strains or partial ruptures, there is thickening of the ligament from edema and hemorrhage, perifascicular edema, and displacement of the ligament fibers from the bony attachment. In grade 3 strains or complete ruptures, there is loss of ligament continuity, disruption of the capsular ligaments, and edema extending to the adjacent subcutaneous fat. There is often an associated joint effusion, and occasionally a "kissing" bone contusion pattern involving the lateral femoral condyle and lateral tibial plateau is produced when these bones, which are opposite to each other, strike together when the MCL ruptures. A complete avulsion of the ligament may give the appearance of a ribbon with an unattached free end and is usually caused by a high-velocity mechanism of injury.

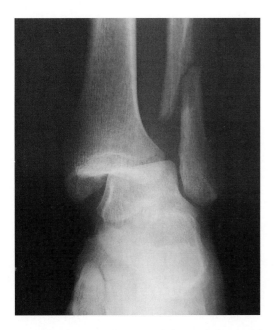 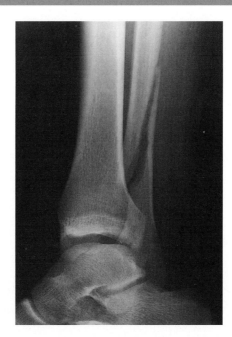

1. What determines stability of the ankle joint?
2. How would you classify this injury using the Lauge-Hansen classification? Using Weber's classification?
3. What is a common mechanism of injury that produces a tibial plafond fracture?
4. How is a mortise projection obtained?

Ankle Fractures (Weber's Classification)

1. The status of the osseous ring (tibia, fibula, and talus), the integrity of the medial and lateral collateral ligaments, and the ligaments of the distal tibiofibular syndesmosis.

2. Type 3 pronation–external rotation. Type C2 Weber.

3. Axial loading (e.g., a fall from height).

4. Anteroposterior view with 15 to 20 degrees of internal rotation of the ankle.

Reference

Hall H: A simplified workable classification of ankle fractures. Foot Ankle 1:5-10, 1980.

Comments

Ankle fractures are frequently complex. Osseous injuries are related to the position of the foot when it is injured and also to the direction of the injury force. Classically, there are four types of injury patterns designated by the Lauge-Hansen classification. The patterns are pronation-abduction, pronation–external rotation, supination-adduction, and supination–external rotation, where the first word identifies the position of the foot and the second word describes the direction of the force. Weber's classification identifies three injury patterns based on the level of a fibular fracture (which is predictive of a syndesmotic injury) and on the degree of displacement of the ankle mortise. In type A injuries, fractures occur below the tibiotalar joint and do not involve the distal tibiofibular syndesmosis. In type B injuries, the fibular fracture occurs at the level of the joint and has an oblique orientation. This injury produces partial disruption of the syndesmosis. There are two type C fractures. Type C1 is characterized by an oblique fibular fracture above the level of the distal tibiofibular ligaments. Type C2 lesions are characterized by an even more proximal fibular fracture, reflecting an extensive rupture of the syndesmosis. Both these injuries are associated with extensive tears of the tibiofibular ligaments. Although Weber's classification does not indicate the mechanism of injury or the full extent of ligament involvement, it correlates well with prognosis and is useful for treatment.

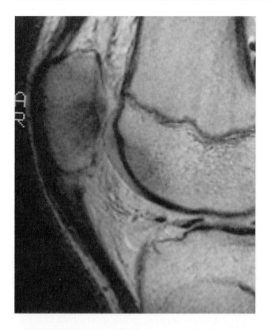
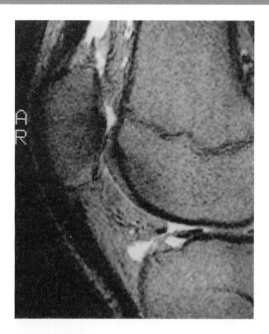
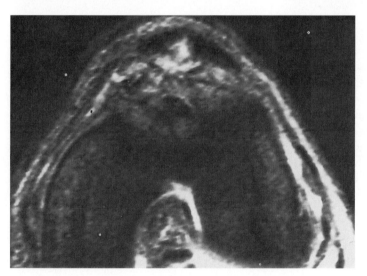

1. Is this condition an inflammatory process?

2. What is meant by "jumper's knee"?

3. What is the most common clinical complaint?

4. What other conditions present with anterior knee pain?

Chronic Patellar Tendinosis (Jumper's Knee)

1. No, it is a degenerative process. There is a conspicuous absence of inflammatory cells when the abnormal tissue is evaluated microscopically.

2. Patellar tendinosis occurs in athletes who participate in activities that require repetitive, violent contraction of the quadriceps musculature, such as basketball and volleyball.

3. Chronic anterior knee pain.

4. Chondromalacia, patellofemoral joint osteoarthritis, crystal deposition arthropathies, osteochondral defect, plica syndrome, Hoffa's syndrome, and prepatellar bursitis.

Reference

Yu JS, Popp JE, Kaeding CC, Lucas J: Correlation of MR imaging and pathologic findings in athletes undergoing surgery for chronic patellar tendinitis. AJR Am J Roentgenol 165:115-118, 1995.

Comments

Patellar tendinosis is caused by repeated microtears occurring at the enthesis of the patellar tendon. Histologically, it is characterized by chronic degeneration, which disrupts the architecture of the tendon. The degree of hyaline degeneration corresponds roughly to the duration of the patient's symptoms and represents an end-stage process. As the disease progresses, it becomes increasingly more difficult to attain pain relief, and the patient experiences diminished athletic performance. In the author's experience, anterior knee pain is best evaluated with magnetic resonance imaging (MRI). Not only is patellar tendinosis easily diagnosed, but so are other conditions that have a similar clinical presentation. The characteristic MRI appearance of patellar tendinosis is focal thickening involving the proximal third of the patellar tendon. The degree of thickening is often two to four times normal tendon thickening. The posterior tendon margin is usually indistinct, and it may be associated with edema in Hoffa's fat pad. Involvement of the anterior fibers does not occur, which can be useful in differentiating tendinosis from acute tears of the proximal patellar tendon. The signal intensity of the tendon is altered with ill-defined areas of intermediate signal intensity on proton density and T2W images. Occasionally, relatively hyperintense signal changes on T2W and short tau inversion recovery images reflect cystic degeneration. The preferred treatment is surgical, with débridement of degenerated tissue and placement of multiple longitudinal tenotomies.

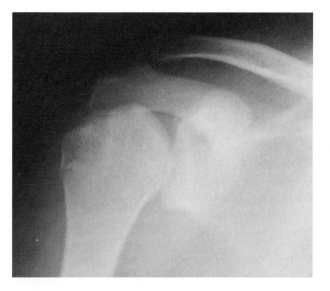
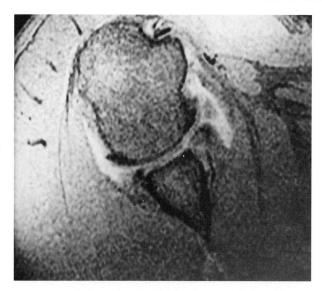

1. What is the finding, and what does it mean?
2. Describe the usual position of the arm when it dislocates anteriorly.
3. What is the main factor that determines a patient's risk for redislocation?
4. Define Bankart's lesion. Does this patient have one?

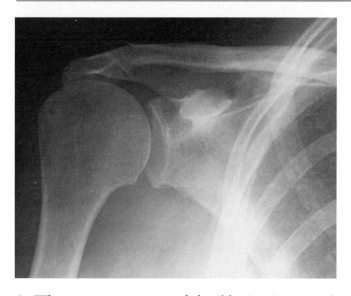
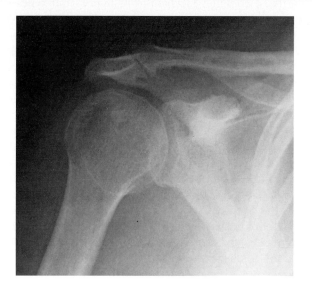

1. What are some causes of shoulder impingement?
2. In this patient, what is the diagnosis, and what is a major contributing factor?
3. What is the aim of treatment?
4. What is the rotator cuff interval? What structure is normally seen here?

Anterior Shoulder Dislocation

1. Hill-Sachs lesion. Anterior glenohumeral dislocation.

2. Hyperabducted, externally rotated, and extended.

3. The age of the patient during the initial dislocation.

4. Avulsion of the anteroinferior labrum by the anterior limb of the inferior glenohumeral ligament with a simultaneous rupture of the anterior periosteum. Yes.

References

Richards RD, Sartoris DJ, Pathria MN, Resnick D: Hill-Sachs lesion and normal humeral groove: MR imaging features allowing their differentiation. Radiology 190:665–668, 1994.

Shankman S, Bencardino J, Beltran J: Glenohumeral instability: Evaluation using MR arthrography of the shoulder. Skeletal Radiol 28:365–382, 1999.

Comments

Approximately 50% of all dislocations in the human body involve the glenohumeral joint. Nearly all these dislocations (95%) result in anterior displacement of the humeral head with respect to the glenoid fossa. An indirect force, such as a fall on an outstretched arm, is the most common mechanism of injury. Four types of anterior dislocations have been described: subcoracoid, subclavicular, subacromial, and intrathoracic. The shoulder must be closely scrutinized for associated injuries after establishing a diagnosis of a dislocation. Impaction fracture of the posterolateral aspect of the humeral head (Hill-Sachs lesion), avulsion of the labrum from the glenoid rim (Bankart's lesion), labra erosion and tear, capsular stripping, and rupture of the subscapularis tendon are common injuries. Radiographically, only the Hill-Sachs lesion and the glenoid rim fracture may be evident. Some have speculated that the size of a Hill-Sachs lesion may be proportional to the length of time that the head has been dislocated, proportional to the number of recurrences, or both. Cross-sectional imaging techniques are useful when the diagnosis is equivocal and for confirming associated injuries to the labrum or labrocapsular complex, such as Bankart's lesion.

Rotator Cuff Tear (Impingement)

1. Conditions that encroach on the subacromial space, such as subacromial spurs, os acromiale, hooked acromial morphology, and acromioclavicular joint osteophytes.

2. Full-thickness rotator cuff tear. Subacromial spur.

3. Restoring the space between the humerus and the coracoacromial arch.

4. The region beneath the coracoacromial arch that is located between the subscapularis and supraspinatus tendons. The intra-articular portion of the long head of the biceps muscle.

References

Jensen KL, Williams GR Jr, Russell IJ, Rockwood CA Jr: Rotator cuff arthropathy. J Bone Joint Surg Am 81:1312–1324, 1999.

Uri DS: MR imaging of shoulder impingement and rotator cuff disease. Radiol Clin North Am 35:77–96, 1997.

Comments

This patient has a full-thickness rotator cuff tear, which allows communication between the glenohumeral joint and the subacromial bursa. Most rotator cuff tears are caused by impingement. Impingement syndrome of the shoulder is a painful condition characterized by sharp pain during abduction and external rotation of the arm or during elevation and internal rotation of the arm. The pathogenesis of this syndrome is related to a loss of space between the proximal humerus and the structures that compose the coracoacromial arch. The region beneath the acromioclavicular joint is also important in impingement. The most vulnerable area of the rotator cuff is the critical zone of the supraspinatus tendon. Subacromial spurs cause mechanical trauma to the musculotendinous junction of the supraspinatus muscle. Degeneration of the cuff often precedes a tear. Another common site of impingement is the rotator cuff interval beneath the coracoacromial arch. Impingement in this location is frequently associated with a hooked acromion process. A third area of impingement is beneath a degenerated acromioclavicular joint and is caused by inferior osteophytosis. In this type of impingement, symptoms occur when the shoulder is abducted more than 120 degrees. On magnetic resonance imaging, effacement of the subacromial fat, with or without subacromial fluid, may be indicative of impingement when it is associated with any of these osseous abnormalities.

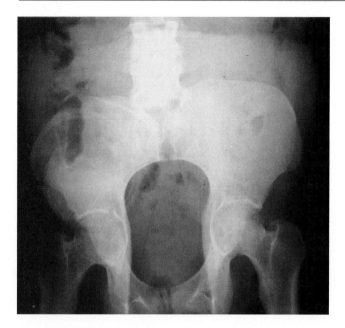

1. What is the diagnosis?
2. What systemic disease did the mother have?
3. List some of the spinal anomalies associated with this condition.
4. What is the VACTERL syndrome, and is it associated with this spine anomaly?

Sacral Agenesis

1. Sacral agenesis (caudal regression syndrome).

2. Diabetes mellitus.

3. Scoliosis, hemivertebra, diastematomyelia, pedicular bar.

4. Complexes associated with anomalies of the *v*ertebral, *a*norectal, *c*ardiac, *t*racheal, *e*sophageal, *r*enal, and *l*imb (musculoskeletal) tissues. Yes.

Reference

Pang D: Sacral agenesis and caudal spinal malformations. Neurosurgery 32:755-778, 1993.

Comments

This case is an "aunt Minnie." The absence of development of a segment of or all of the lumbar spine and sacrum is a rare condition. Complete absence of the sacrum occurs in about 30% of patients with sacral agenesis. The radiographic findings are characteristic. There is usually incomplete development of the sacrum, although one or more segments may be present. In the absence of the sacrum, the ilia articulate with the lumbar spine, drawing these bones to the midline so that the pelvis appears narrowed. Scoliosis is common (more than 50% of cases), as are spinal anomalies. Urinary incontinence or dysfunction from bladder and upper urinary tract anomalies is a common finding. Dural sac stenosis and a low conus medullaris with tethering of the cord may be present, which is often associated with an anterior sacral meningocele.

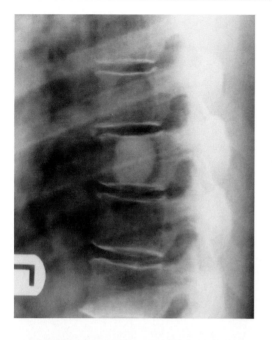
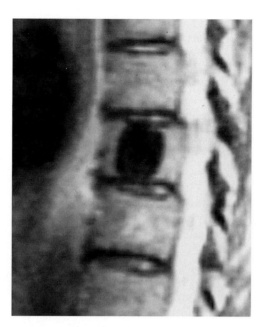
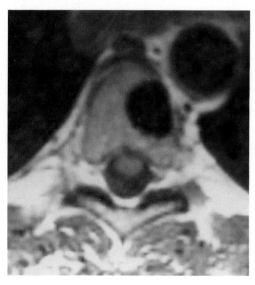

1. What diagnoses would you consider in this patient?
2. Can a bone island enlarge? In whom is this more likely to occur?
3. Is it unusual for this lesion to show scintigraphic activity?
4. What is osteopoikilosis?

Vertebral Enostosis

1. Large enostosis, osteoid osteoma, solitary osteoma, metastasis, and low-grade infection.

2. Yes. Adolescents during periods of growth.

3. Yes, but it can occur when the lesion is large or if it is imaged during new bone formation.

4. A condition characterized by multiple enostosis, usually in a periarticular distribution.

Reference

Murphey MD, Andrews CL, Flemming DJ, et al: From the archives of the AFIP. Primary tumors of the spine: Radiologic pathologic correlation. Radiographics 16:1131–1158, 1996.

Comments

A vertebral enostosis, or bone island, occurs in 1% to 14% of all spines. Generally, the lesions are quite small and have a characteristic appearance—a small, sclerotic focus within the medullary cavity of a vertebral body that is histologically identical to lamellar bone. These lesions are most common in the thoracic and lumbar spine and may have a variety of shapes. Although the majority of enostoses are small and inconspicuous, on occasion, these lesions may become quite large, demonstrate scintigraphic activity, and even show growth. Under these situations, it may be difficult to exclude metastasis, and you may need to biopsy a lesion to exclude a neoplastic process. The radiographic appearance of a bone island is typically a dense, solitary, sclerotic lesion located close to a vertebral margin. Generally, lesions are well defined but contain spiculated margins that are conspicuous on computed tomography. On magnetic resonance imaging, an enostosis demonstrates uniform low signal intensity throughout the lesion on all pulse sequences and no peritumoral edema or pathologic enhancement.

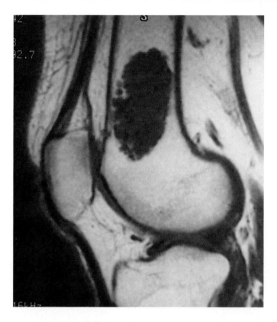 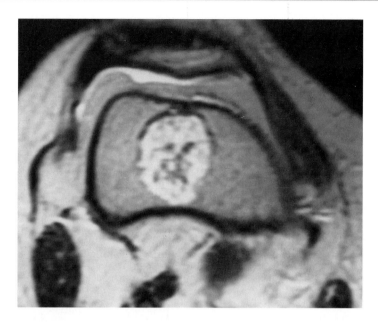

1. Can this neoplasm undergo malignant transformation? Into what?

2. Where is a common location for this neoplasm in the hands and feet?

3. What are some radiographic indicators of malignant transformation? Is location helpful in predicting risk?

4. What is the differential diagnosis of a phalangeal enchondroma?

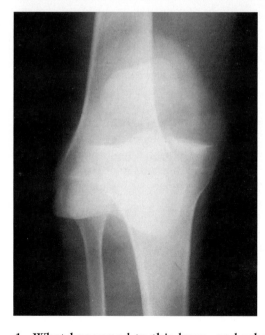 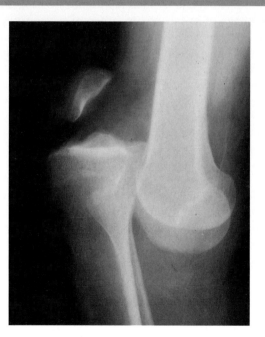

1. What happened to this knee, and what is the most critical step in the evaluation of this extremity?

2. How are these injuries classified?

3. Which is worse, an anterior or a posterior dislocation?

4. What does a foot drop indicate? Is this injury permanent?

Enchondroma

1. Yes. Chondrosarcoma, malignant fibrohistiocytoma, fibrosarcoma, and osteosarcoma have been reported.

2. In the diaphysis of the short tubular bones (phalanges and metacarpals).

3. Enlarging osteolytic area, development of pathologic fracture or soft-tissue mass, and disappearance of an existing calcification. Yes, proximal lesions are more likely to degenerate.

4. Giant cell tumor, aneurysmal bone cyst, solitary bone cyst, and fibrous dysplasia.

Reference

Mandell GA, Harcke HT, Kumar SJ: Chondroid lesions of the extremities. Top Magn Reson Imaging 4:56–65, 1991.

Comments

An enchondroma is a cartilaginous tumor that arises within the medullary cavity of a bone. It is composed of lobules of hyaline cartilage and is thought to originate from a cartilage rest that has become displaced from the growth plate. Characteristically, it is discovered in the third or fourth decade of life. Generally, enchondromas are asymptomatic and are detected as incidental findings. The appearance of pain may indicate malignant transformation. Nearly 50% of enchondromas are found in the small tubular bones of the hand. In order of decreasing frequency, enchondromas affect the proximal phalanges, metacarpal bones, middle phalanges, and distal phalanges. Long tubular bones are affected in 25% of cases and occur more frequently in the upper than in the lower extremity. Involvement of the axial skeleton is rare.

This patient shows a typical magnetic resonance appearance of an enchondroma. Solitary enchondromas are usually centrally located. These lesions are well defined, often with a lobulated contour, and frequently contain stippled calcifications. They demonstrate homogeneous low signal intensity on T1W images and fairly homogeneous high signal intensity on T2W images, except in areas of calcifications. Endosteal scalloping may occur if the lesion is eccentrically located. Occasionally, it may have an expansile configuration with a thinned cortex. Periostitis and cortical breakthrough are not features of an enchondroma.

Complete Knee Dislocation

1. Complete knee dislocation. Assess the vascular supply for injuries, particularly intimal tears of the popliteal artery.

2. By the position of the tibia relative to the femur.

3. A posterior dislocation tends to cause more soft-tissue injuries, including tears of cruciate and collateral ligaments, meniscal tears, and frequent ruptures of the popliteus complex.

4. An injury to the common peroneal nerve. Usually.

Reference

Yu JS, Goodwin D, Salonen D, et al: Complete dislocation of the knee: Spectrum of associated soft-tissue injuries depicted by MR imaging. AJR Am J Roentgenol 164:135–139, 1995.

Comments

A dislocation of the knee is a severe injury that is caused by high-energy trauma. The incidence of complete knee dislocations is reportedly low, although any estimate is speculative because many dislocations reduce spontaneously at the scene of the injury. Therefore, a patient who had a knee dislocation may present with extensive ligamentous disruption without an obvious dislocation. There are five types of knee dislocations: anterior, posterior, lateral, medial, and posterolateral. Anterior and posterior dislocations account for the majority of dislocations. Both cruciate ligaments are likely to be torn, although, in certain situations, the posterior cruciate ligament may be spared. Injuries involving both collateral ligaments and menisci are common. Injury to the popliteal tendon denotes a more severe mechanism of injury and is likely to be the result of posterior or posterolateral dislocations. A knee dislocation constitutes a true orthopedic emergency owing to the possibility of associated injuries to the popliteal artery or the common peroneal nerve. Vascular injuries occur in 33% to 40% of patients, and up to 50% of patients require an amputation when vascular lesions are not treated promptly. An emergent lower extremity angiogram to assess the vascular supply is recommended, even if a pulse is palpable in the foot, because latent thrombosis may occur from an unsuspected intimal injury. Peroneal nerve injuries may occur in 14% to 35% of patients and usually cause a permanent defect.

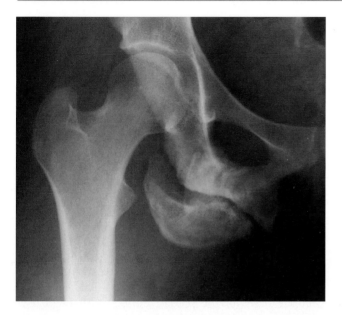

1. A former athlete presented with this radiograph. Describe the findings.
2. How would the athlete have presented?
3. If symptoms persisted but radiographs remained normal, what would you recommend, and why?
4. Would you recommend a biopsy?

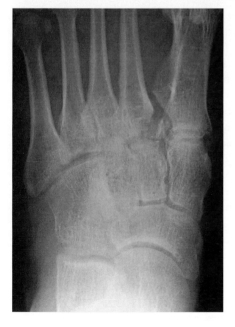
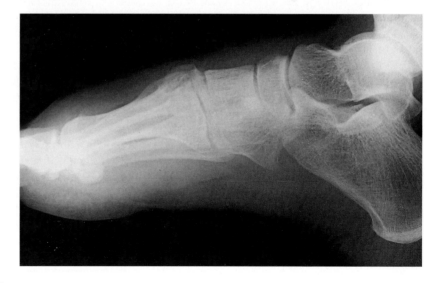

1. What is the mechanism of injury?
2. Name the different types of tarsometatarsal dislocation patterns. What type does this patient have?
3. If you suspect this injury, but the initial radiographic series is equivocal, what simple maneuver can you perform to stress the foot?
4. What vascular structure may be injured in Lisfranc's fracture-dislocation?

C A S E 3 3

Avulsion of the Ischial Tuberosity

1. Avulsion of the right ischial tuberosity ossification center.

2. Acute pain and swelling in the groin or near the hip joint.

3. Magnetic resonance imaging, because it is capable of demonstrating injuries to ligaments and tendons that are not apparent radiographically.

4. No.

Reference

Fernbach SK, Wilkinson RH: Avulsion injuries of the pelvis and proximal femur. AJR Am J Roentgenol 137:581–584, 1984.

Comments

Avulsion injuries about the pelvis are not uncommon in the adolescent or young adult athlete. Activities associated with such injuries include those that require repetitive to-and-fro adduction and abduction or flexion and extension. Hurdlers, sprinters, and cheerleaders are especially susceptible to this type of injury, largely owing to the stresses experienced at the origin and insertion sites of different muscle groups during this activity. An avulsion of the ischial tuberosity ossification center, the attachment of the hamstring muscle group, is one such injury. It is common in hurdlers. An avulsion of the rectus femoris muscle origin is another such injury, often heralded by the presence of small flecks of bone adjacent to the superior acetabular rim (reflected head) or in the region of the inferior anterior iliac spine (straight head). Other common potential sites of avulsion in the pelvis and hips include the anterior superior iliac spine (origin of the sartorius muscle or tensor fasciae femoris), the apophysis of the lesser trochanter (insertion of the psoas muscle), the greater trochanter (insertion of the gluteal musculature), the apophysis of the iliac crest (insertion of the abdominal musculature), and the parasymphyseal region of the pubis (origin of the adductor muscles). The radiographic hallmark of avulsion injuries is irregularity of the cortex at the site of avulsion and displaced pieces of bone of variable size. Follow-up radiographs may reveal hypertrophic new bone formation, which can be associated with marked skeletal overgrowth or deformity, mimicking a neoplasm (as in this case).

C A S E 3 4

Lisfranc's Fracture-Dislocation

1. Forced plantar flexion of the forefoot.

2. Homolateral, partial incongruity, and divergent Lisfranc's fracture-dislocation. Partial incongruity.

3. Perform a standing lateral view to look for dorsal displacement of the metatarsal bones.

4. The dorsalis pedis artery.

Reference

Norfray JF, Geline RA, Steinberg RI, et al: Subtleties of Lisfranc fracture-dislocations. AJR Am J Roentgenol 137:1151–1156, 1981.

Comments

Tarsometatarsal fracture-dislocations are also known as Lisfranc's injuries. Transverse metatarsal ligaments connect the bases of the second through fifth metatarsal bones, but this ligament does not exist between the first and second metatarsal bones. Instead, the base of the second metatarsal bone is attached to the medial cuneiform by an oblique ligament (Lisfranc's ligament). Avulsion fractures of the second metatarsal base frequently occur at the enthesis of this ligament. Because there is greater support on the plantar surface by the plantar ligaments and tendons, most dislocations occur dorsally.

Lisfranc's injuries may have several patterns. A homolateral (convergent) pattern occurs when there is displacement of all five metatarsal bases, and the direction of displacement is nearly always laterally. A partial incongruity pattern occurs when there is a fracture of the first metatarsal base with displacement of the shaft medially, or when there is lateral displacement of the second to fifth metatarsals. A divergent pattern occurs when the first metatarsal base displaces medially without a fracture and the second metatarsal or a combination of the second to fifth metatarsals displaces laterally. Treatment is aimed at restoring the anatomy. If displacement is less than 2 mm, closed reduction is adequate. More significant fracture-dislocations require open reduction and internal fixation. If reduction is difficult, evaluation with magnetic resonance imaging or computed tomography is advocated to exclude entrapment of either a tendon or a fracture fragment.

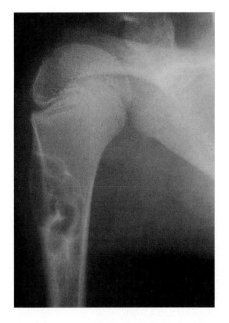
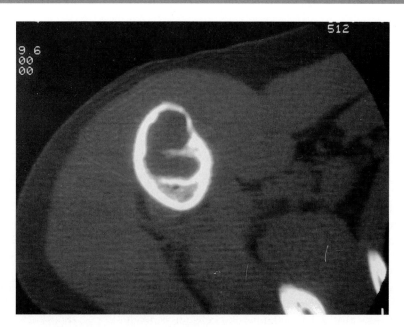

1. List your differential diagnoses (keep in mind the age of the patient).

2. Which of the lesions from this list can appear very aggressive and mimic a malignant neoplasm?

3. Which malignant neoplasm can mimic an aneurysmal bone cyst?

4. What is the estimated incidence of fibrous cortical defects in children older than 2 years? In people 20 years old?

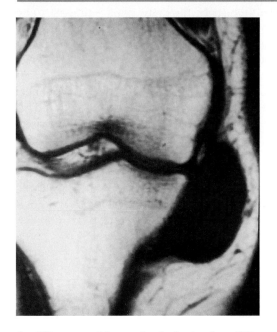
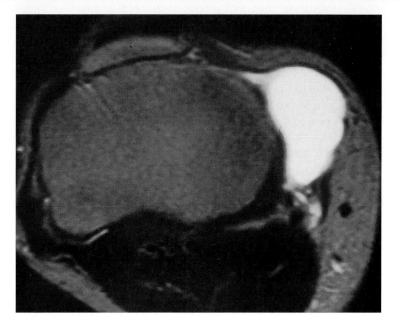

1. What would you include in the differential diagnosis?

2. What is the cause of pes anserine bursitis?

3. Can you make a diagnosis of a meniscal cyst if you do not identify a meniscal tear?

4. How is a meniscal cyst treated? What if you were to only aspirate it?

Nonossifying Fibroma

1. Nonossifying fibroma, eosinophilic granuloma (EG), aneurysmal bone cyst, fibrous dysplasia, osteoblastoma, chondromyxoid fibroma, and desmoplastic fibroma.

2. Desmoplastic fibroma and EG.

3. Telangiectatic osteogenic sarcoma.

4. Between 20% and 50%. About 2%.

Reference

Jee WH, Choe BY, Kang HS, et al: Nonossifying fibroma: Characteristics at MR imaging with pathologic correlation. Radiology 209:197–202, 1998.

Comments

Nonossifying fibroma is a benign lesion of bone characterized by bundles of spindle-shaped connective tissue cells, giant cells, and xanthomatous cells. It is likely derived from the proliferation of a fibrous cortical defect into the medullary space. It presents in the first and second decades of life, is often incidentally detected, and may undergo spontaneous regression. Most lesions occur in the metadiaphyseal region of a long bone of the lower extremity, eccentrically located in the bone.

The radiographic appearance of a nonossifying fibroma is not very specific. A description of a multiloculated, radiolucent lesion varying from 2 cm to 7 cm, oriented along the long axis of the bone, with a well-defined rim of sclerosis, and demonstrating scalloped margins (that can expand the bone) can apply to a number of lesions. In skeletally immature patients, the location of the "soap bubble" lesion can be helpful. If it is centrally located, think simple bone cyst, aneurysmal bone cyst, and desmoplastic fibroma, while the other lesions in the differential are more eccentrically located. All of them can involve the metaphysis of the bone, so if it extends toward the diaphysis, think nonossifying fibroma, simple bone cyst, and osteoblastoma. Aneurysmal bone cyst, giant cell tumor, chondromyxoid fibroma, and desmoplastic fibroma extend to the epiphysis. EG and fibrous dysplasia can look like anything. And, let's face it, chondromyxoid fibroma, osteoblastoma (appendicular), and desmoplastic fibroma are so uncommon, they should not be your top three choices.

Meniscal Cyst

1. Meniscal cyst, ganglion cyst, synovial cyst, and—less likely—pes anserine bursitis.

2. The anserine bursa becomes inflamed when it is traumatized from repeated flexion, extension, and rotation of the knee.

3. Yes, because only 60% to 85% of cysts have an identifiable meniscal tear.

4. Repair or débride the meniscal tear. The cyst would recur.

References

Burk DL, Dalinka MK, Kanal E, et al: Meniscal and ganglion cysts of the knee: MR evaluation. AJR Am J Roentgenol 150:331–336, 1988.

Coral A, van Holsbeeck M, Adler RS: Imaging of meniscal cyst of the knee in three cases. Skeletal Radiol 18:451–455, 1989.

Comments

The clinical symptoms of a meniscal cyst vary, although joint line pain associated with a palpable mass is a classic presentation. The incidence of meniscal cysts has been reported to be between 1% and 2% in knees that undergo a diagnostic study. A meniscal cyst is caused by decompression of synovial fluid through a meniscal tear. Stretching of the knee capsule and parameniscal soft tissues by the cystic mass is thought to be the cause of the pain. Most patients are in their third or fourth decade of life when first evaluated, and men are more frequently affected than are women. These cysts are common after meniscectomy, trauma, or significant degeneration of a meniscus. When a tear is horizontally oriented, it is more likely to communicate with a cyst. Remember that three fourths of these cysts are palpable. One important clue to the diagnosis is that the size of the meniscal cyst may increase and decrease with different knee positions. Long-standing cysts may be large, may contain extruded meniscal debris, and may cause erosive changes in the adjacent tibial cortex.

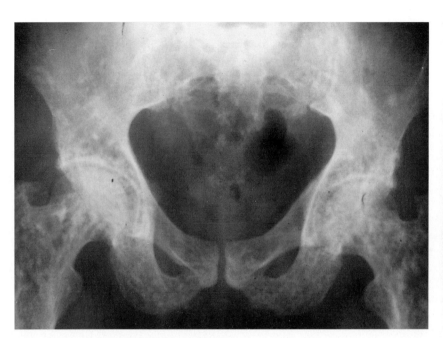

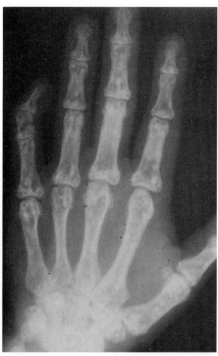

1. Is there a differential diagnosis?
2. What is a common cutaneous lesion associated with this disorder, and how frequently is it seen?
3. What other disorders have an association with this condition?
4. What does each lesion represent histologically?

Osteopoikilosis

1. Not in this case, but occasionally epiphyseal dysplasia, melorheostosis, osteoblastic metastasis, and—rarely—sclerotic forms of multiple myeloma and sarcoidosis can be diagnosed.

2. Dermatofibrosis lenticularis disseminata. Twenty-five percent of cases.

3. Scleroderma, cleft palate, dwarfism, syndactyly, endocrine disorders, melorheostosis, and dystocia.

4. A focus of lamellar bone containing haversian systems.

Reference

Lagier R, Mbakop A, Bigler A: Osteopoikilosis: A radiological and pathological study. Skeletal Radiol 11:161–168, 1984.

Comments

Osteopoikilosis is a rare bone dysplasia characterized by the presence of numerous round or oval foci of compact bone within the spongiosa. The etiology is unknown, although a familial occurrence has been reported and it is believed to be transmitted as an autosomal dominant disorder. This disorder may become evident at any age and has no sexual predilection. Clinically, the manifestations are usually mild or absent. The radiographic findings in this case are characteristic of osteopoikilosis. Small, numerous, well-defined areas of sclerosis measuring a few millimeters to several centimeters in size are the principal finding. These lesions tend to cluster in a periarticular distribution with a predilection for the epiphysis and metaphysis of a bone. Lesions also commonly involve the carpus, tarsus, pelvis, and scapula. Involvement of the skull, clavicle, ribs, mandible, sternum, and vertebral bodies is unusual. Bone scintigraphy usually shows no radionuclide uptake except on rare occasions. The differential diagnosis is limited when you consider the symmetrical distribution, clustering about the joints, and uniformity of size of lesions, which are distinctive features not present in other disorders.

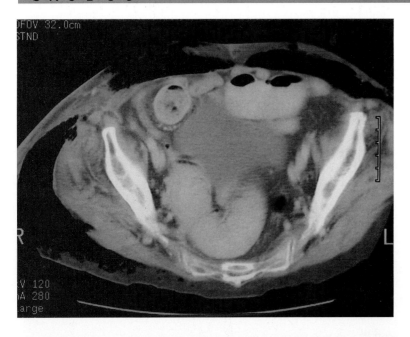

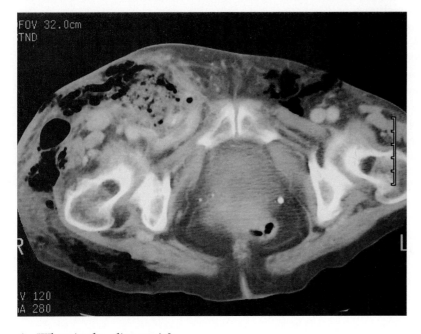

1. What is the diagnosis?

2. What should be done next?

3. What is the most common infectious agent in pyomyositis? What muscles are affected?

4. Subcutaneous emphysema and pneumomediastinum should alert you to what condition?

Gas Gangrene

1. Gas gangrene from a visceral perforation.

2. Surgical débridement and repair of the bowel perforation.

3. *Staphylococcus aureus.* Large muscle groups, particularly those of the lower extremity.

4. Rupture of the trachea or main bronchus.

Reference

Yu JS: MR imaging of soft tissue trauma. Emerg Radiol 3:181–194, 1996.

Comments

In this case, the observed finding is straightforward—gas in the soft tissue. The cause, however, requires a little bit of thought. The appearance of gas in the soft tissues is quite distinctive owing to the radiolucency that gas creates. Causes of gas in the soft tissues include iatrogenic infiltration of air, gas gangrene, abscess, and pyomyositis. Air infiltration can occur with rib fractures (pneumothorax), tracheostomy (pneumomediastinum), and thoracotomy (subcutaneous emphysema). Rupture of the trachea or main bronchus can be an acute source of pneumomediastinum and subcutaneous emphysema in the setting of trauma. A gas phlegmon is created by an infection. Debilitated people can develop a gangrenous infection when there is a visceral perforation or a communicating viscerocutaneous sinus tract from ulceration of the gastrointestinal tract. Immunosuppression with corticosteroid medication or chemotherapy agents often contributes to the insidious nature of the infection. Suppurative bacterial myositis, or pyomyositis, is a condition caused by bacterial infection that develops in the larger muscle groups of the thigh after minor trauma. Ninety percent of cases are caused by *S. aureus.* Chronic steroid use or an underlying disease such as diabetes, acquired immunodeficiency syndrome, connective tissue disorders, or malignancy is considered a predisposing condition.

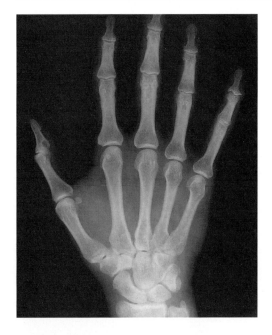

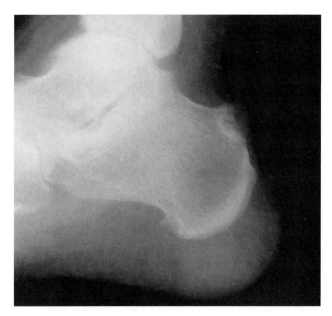

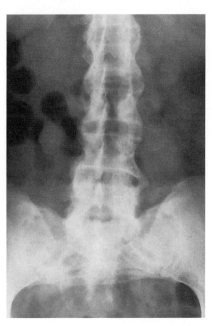

1. What are some characteristic findings of this disease process in the hands and feet?

2. About 2% to 6% of patients with psoriasis are affected with an arthropathy. Who is at risk?

3. What percentage of people with psoriatic skin disease develop sacroiliac joint abnormalities? What percentage of patients with psoriatic arthropathy develop sacroiliac joint abnormalities?

4. What differentiates the paravertebral ossification of this disease from syndesmophytes in patients with ankylosing spondylitis?

Psoriatic Arthritis

1. Soft-tissue swelling, joint space narrowing, erosions with accompanying bony proliferation, "pencil-in-cup" osteolysis.

2. Patients with moderate to severe skin abnormalities; the strongest association is with patients who demonstrate nail changes.

3. About 10% to 25% with psoriatic skin disease and 30% to 50% with arthropathy.

4. Does not involve the annulus fibrosus.

Reference

El-Khoury GY, Kathol MH, Brandser EA: Seronegative spondyloarthropathies. Radiol Clin North Am 34:343-357, 1996.

Comments

Psoriatic arthritis is a synovial inflammatory arthropathy that is considered a seronegative rheumatoid variant. It generally affects patients with moderate to severe skin disease, but its strongest correlation is with patients who demonstrate nail abnormalities such as pitting, ridging, splintering, and thickening. This arthropathy has five presentations: distal interphalangeal joint polyarthritis, arthritis mutilans, rheumatoid arthritis–like symmetrical polyarthritis, monoarthritis or asymmetrical oligoarthritis, and sacroiliitis and spondylitis mimicking ankylosing spondylitis. The arthropathy may antedate skin changes in 20% of cases. The radiographic hallmark of this disease is bone proliferation, distinguishing it from rheumatoid arthritis (the prototypical non–bone-forming synovial inflammatory arthropathy). The joints of the hands and feet are common target sites. Key observations include soft-tissue swelling that sometimes involves the entire digit ("sausage finger"); normal mineralization; bony erosions that begin at the margins of the joint and progress centrally, destroying the entire articular surface area (pencil-in-cup deformity); and resorption of the tufts of the distal phalanges. Bony proliferative changes tend to occur adjacent to these erosions but may also occur in the form of periostitis, joint ankylosis, and enthesopathy. In the axial skeleton, bilateral sacroiliitis is more frequent than is unilateral involvement and may be either symmetrical or asymmetrical. In the spine, asymmetrical or unilateral paravertebral ossifications affect the lower thoracic and upper lumbar spine.

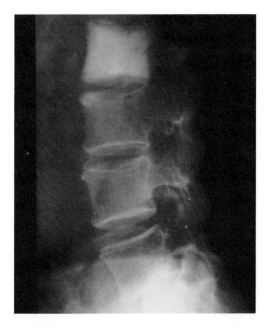

1. List your differential considerations.

2. What neoplasms can cause osteoblastic metastasis?

3. Which disease is associated with the "sandwich vertebra" sign?

4. How is fluorosis different radiographically from the other conditions that depict diffusely increased bone density?

Ivory Vertebra

1. Osteoblastic metastasis, lymphoma, Paget's disease, chronic infection, and—occasionally—osteosarcoma.

2. Pure osteoblastic lesions—prostate carcinoma; common osteoblastic lesions—bronchial carcinoid tumor, medulloblastoma, neuroblastoma, and carcinomas of the breast, bladder, nasopharynx, and stomach; occasional osteoblastic lesions—chordoma, lymphoma, and multiple myeloma.

3. Osteopetrosis tarda, which refers to increased density occurring at the end plates.

4. Development of prominent, densely sclerotic osteophytes, which project into the paravertebral soft tissues at the attachment of ligaments, tendons, and muscle.

Reference

Silverman IE, Flynn JA: Images in clinical medicine. Ivory vertebra. N Engl J Med 338:100, 1998.

Comments

Metastasis is the most common tumor of the spine. Metastasis to the axial skeleton occurs in nearly half of patients who have been discovered to have osseous metastasis on bone scintigraphy, most frequently involving the thoracic and lumbar vertebral bodies. When a vertebral body is heterogeneously or homogeneously sclerotic, it is referred to as an *ivory vertebra*. When the process is more diffuse, affecting numerous vertebral bodies, other conditions, such as mastocytosis, tuberous sclerosis, myelofibrosis, renal osteodystrophy, fluorosis, and osteopetrosis, should be considered.

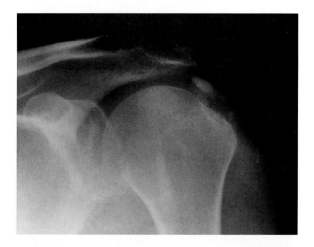
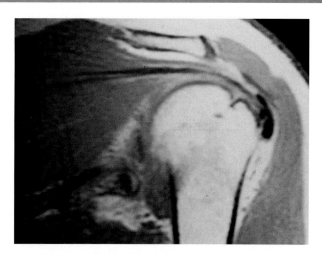
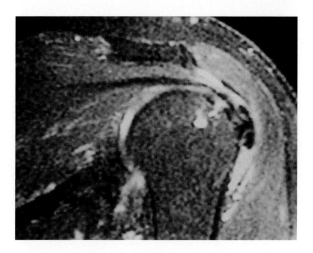

1. Are patients more likely to be symptomatic when the calcifications are ill defined or when they are sharply defined?

2. Once a calcification is identified, does it ever change in appearance?

3. What percentage of people with periarticular calcifications are symptomatic?

4. What pathologic cascade causes structural damage in the joint?

Calcific Tendinitis and Bursitis

1. Ill-defined calcifications indicate calcium resorption, the active phase of the disease.

2. Yes, frequently these calcifications may be resorbed, become denser, increase in size, or change in position.

3. About 33%.

4. Hydroxyapatite crystals are released into the synovial fluid, which becomes engulfed by fixed, macrophage-like synovial cells that release the enzymes collagenase and protease, which attack the periarticular tissues, including the rotator cuff, which destabilizes the joint, causing progressive joint destruction, which releases more crystals into the fluid.

Reference

Ishii H, Brunet JA, Welsh RP, Uhthoff HK: "Bursal reactions" in rotator cuff tearing, the impingement syndrome, and calcifying tendinitis. J Shoulder Elbow Surg 6:131–136, 1997.

Comments

Calcific tendinitis and subdeltoid bursitis are two manifestations of a spectrum of conditions caused by the deposition of calcium hydroxyapatite crystals in the soft tissues. The shoulder joint is the articulation most commonly involved, although virtually any joint may be affected. Periarticular deposits of these crystals are often asymptomatic, but when they are associated with acute inflammation, patients complain of severe pain, swelling, occasional erythema, and fever, as with a septic joint.

Deposits consisting of granular inclusions of calcium hydroxyapatite are associated with necrosis and inflammation. Radiographically, these deposits appear ill defined and cloudlike initially but become denser and more sharply defined. Ill-defined deposits show histologic evidence of calcium resorption and correlate with symptomatic episodes. The insertion of the supraspinatus tendon is the most frequent site involved. Structural damage can produce degenerative changes in the joint and rotator cuff defects. Radiographic findings include loss of joint space, destruction of bone, subchondral sclerosis, intra-articular debris, and joint disorganization. Rotator cuff tears cause superior migration of the humeral head, which often contacts the inferior surface of the acromion process. Because these deposits may become extruded from the tendon into the surrounding bursa, tendinitis and bursitis can coexist in the joint.

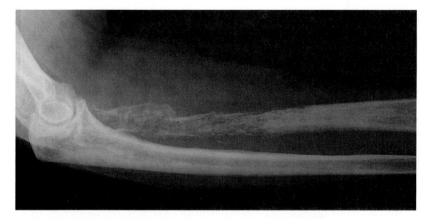

1. List the three main patterns of bone destruction.

2. What pattern is shown in this patient? What are the processes that can cause this particular pattern of bone destruction?

3. What mechanisms allow the spread of tumor to bone?

4. List the most common tumor of origin for bone metastasis in adult men, adult women, and children.

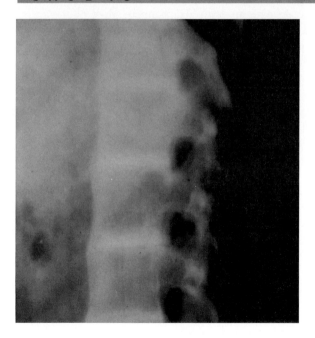

1. What is your differential diagnosis?

2. Homogentisic acid oxidase is an active participant in what metabolic pathways?

3. What processes can cause discal calcifications?

4. What differentiates the peripheral arthropathy of this condition from ankylosing spondylitis?

Permeative Bone Destruction

1. Geographic, moth eaten, and permeative.

2. Permeative pattern—metastasis, primary bone tumors (e.g., Ewing's sarcoma), multiple myeloma, leukemia, eosinophilic granuloma, and osteomyelitis.

3. Direct extension, lymphatic spread, hematogenous spread, and intraspinal spread.

4. Adult men: prostate, lung, and bladder; adult women: breast and uterus; children: neuroblastoma, Ewing's sarcoma, osteosarcoma, and soft-tissue tumors.

Reference

Lodwick GS: Solitary malignant tumors of bone: The application of predictor variables in diagnosis. Semin Roentgenol 1:293-313, 1966.

Comments

There are three basic patterns of bone destruction: geographic, a marginated or circumscribed solitary area of bone lysis; moth eaten, caused by numerous smaller osteolytic lesions and endosteal excavations generally indicating a more aggressive lesion; and permeative, an aggressive infiltrative process that causes cortical tunneling, numerous tiny and indistinct osteolytic lesions with poor margination between abnormal and normal bone. This patient has breast cancer and demonstrates a good example of a permeative pattern of bone destruction from an osseous metastasis. However, there are many causes of permeative bone lesions, including both benign and malignant processes, so it is important to search for other clues that can aid in narrowing the differential diagnosis, such as age of the patient, presence of other lesions, soft-tissue involvement, underlying systemic disease, and constitutional signs (fever, elevated white blood cell count).

Ochronosis (Alkaptonuria)

1. Ochronosis, ankylosing spondylitis, dystrophic calcifications in the disk, calcium pyrophosphate dihydrate (CPPD) crystal deposition disease.

2. Phenylalanine and tyrosine.

3. Ochronosis, CPPD crystal deposition disease, hemochromatosis, hyperparathyroidism, acromegaly, poliomyelitis, amyloidosis, and spinal fusion.

4. It does not involve the small joints of the hands and feet.

Reference

Hamdi N, Cooke TD, Hassan B: Ochronotic arthropathy: Case report and review of the literature. Int Orthop 23:122-125, 1999.

Comments

The keys to the correct diagnosis in this case, which has a very similar appearance to a "bamboo spine," are the discal calcifications. Ochronosis is a rare, inherited disorder characterized by pigmentation of connective tissue in patients with alkaptonuria. Most patients present in the second or third decades of life, and there is a 2:1 male predilection. It is an inborn metabolic disorder caused by the absence of homogentisic acid oxidase, resulting in excessive production and deposition of homogentisic acid in cartilage and other connective tissue. This pigmentation then leads to degeneration and calcification. Patients are more frequently symptomatic from spondylosis than from the peripheral arthropathy caused by this disease.

The radiographic findings shown in this case are classic. The most common location in the vertebral column is the lumbar spine, followed by the thoracic and cervical spine. Calcification of the disk is laminated, often sparing the central region, and composed of calcium hydroxyapatite. Degenerative changes develop with disk space narrowing and end plate osteophytosis, and the bone density becomes diminished. The presence of vacuum phenomena at numerous levels is not uncommon, and there is often a loss of lumbar lordosis. Peripheral joints commonly affected include shoulder, hip, and knee joints. In these joints, calcified loose bodies are common.

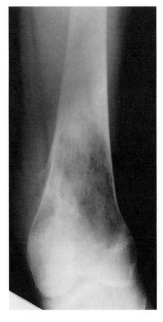

1. What is the likely diagnosis? What would you do next?
2. Can this tumor occur in the diaphysis of a tubular bone?
3. Describe a telangiectatic osteosarcoma.
4. What is the characteristic location and pattern of periostitis of a periosteal osteosarcoma?

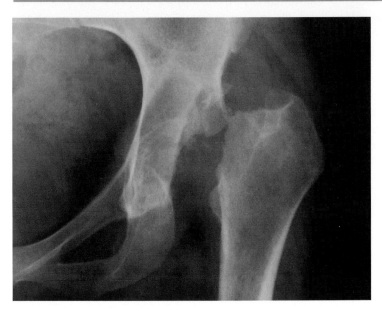

1. What is your differential diagnosis?
2. In the United States, what is the most common cause of a Lisfranc fracture-dislocation–like appearance of the foot?
3. Which diseases are most likely to cause the changes depicted in this patient?
4. List the characteristic radiographic features of the hypertrophic form of this condition.

Osteogenic Sarcoma

1. Conventional osteosarcoma. Computed tomography or magnetic resonance imaging of the femur to determine the extent of the lesion, biopsy, and then staging of the patient.

2. Yes, although fewer than 10% do.

3. An osteolytic subtype of osteosarcoma that may appear benign, mimicking an aneurysmal bone cyst or giant cell tumor.

4. Diaphyseal and juxtacortical—radiating osseous spicules that extend from the superficial region of the cortex into the adjacent soft tissue, often in a perpendicular orientation to the cortex.

Reference

Murphey MD, Robbin MR, McRae GA, et al: The many faces of osteosarcoma. Radiographics 17:1205-1231, 1997.

Comments

This case is straightforward. There is a large lytic mass in the distal femoral metaphysis associated with Codman's triangle, a prominent triangular area of periosteal new bone at the margin of the tumor. There is a wide zone of transition and an aggressive, moth-eaten appearance. The key observation is the presence of an osseous matrix in the medial aspect of the tumor, producing variable density in the involved portion of the distal femur. Osteosarcoma is the most common primary malignant neoplasm of bone in adolescents and young adults. The most common clinical presentation is pain at the tumor site. It usually begins as an insidious pain but progresses to become severe and constant. The development of a palpable soft-tissue mass or a pathologic fracture is also a common presentation. Although an osseous matrix characterizes this tumor, the radiographic appearance can range from densely blastic to nearly completely lytic. Osteoid can also be formed from cartilaginous tissue, which is often present in abundance in this tumor. Only 50% of tumors produce sufficient osteoid to be termed osteoblastic, whereas 25% produce predominantly cartilage (chondroblastic), and 25% produce predominantly spindle cells (fibroblastic).

Neuroarthropathy (Atrophic Type)

1. Atrophic neuroarthropathy, massive Gorham's osteolysis, posttraumatic osteolysis, metastasis, tumor, and infection.

2. Diabetes mellitus.

3. Tabes dorsalis or syringomyelia.

4. Recall the "five Ds": increased density, joint distention, intra-articular and periarticular debris, joint disorganization, and dislocation.

Reference

Yu JS: Diabetic foot and neuroarthropathy: Magnetic resonance imaging features. Top Magn Reson Imaging 9:295-310, 1998.

Comments

Neuropathic osteoarthropathy, or neuroarthropathy, is a complex complication of neuropathic disease. The pathogenesis of neuropathic disorders remains debatable, but many experts consider repetitive trauma and altered sympathetic control of blood flow to be significant factors. Loss of the protective sensations of pain and proprioception leads to chronic destabilization of the joint. The resultant changes in the articular cartilage cause fibrillation and degeneration, and eventual erosion of the cortical surfaces. Neuroarthropathy has three presentations; hypertrophic, atrophic, and mixed. In atrophic neuroarthropathy, there is resorption of the bone producing a well-demarcated transition between the lysed and remaining bone. Several important observations in this patient are notable. There is no evidence of a fracture or of accompanying bone repair, the bone density at the margin of lysis is normal, and there is no indication of surgery. This presentation of neuroarthropathy is much more common in the upper extremity and is usually associated with syringomyelia or peripheral nerve injury. In the lower extremity, the hip and the knee are common locations, and neuroarthropathy here is more likely to be caused by either tabes dorsalis or syringomyelia. In the hip, soft-tissue swelling (notice the displaced capsular and gluteal fat stripes), caused by an effusion and capsular hypertrophy, and intra-articular debris are important clues to diagnosis.

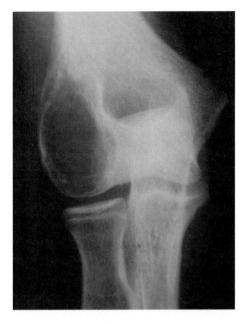
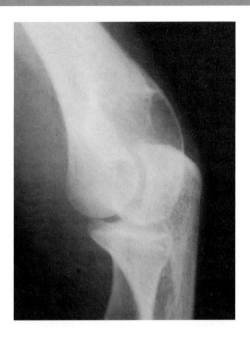

1. List your differential diagnoses.

2. What is a potential complication of this tumor after it has been irradiated?

3. This tumor is rare in the skull unless it is accompanied by what disorder?

4. On magnetic resonance imaging, a low signal intensity rim often surrounds this lesion. What causes this appearance?

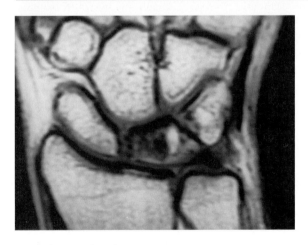
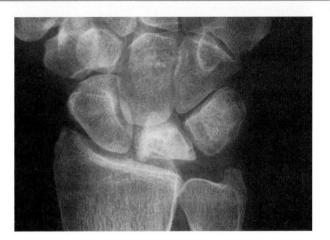

1. What is the diagnosis?

2. Can the process be interrupted with treatment?

3. Does the length of the ulna contribute to the disease process?

4. What is the preferred method of diagnosing fractures of the lunate?

Giant Cell Tumor

1. Giant cell tumor (GCT); aneurysmal bone cyst; chondroblastoma; brown tumor of hyperparathyroidism; and, occasionally, chondromyxoid fibroma.

2. Malignant transformation into an osteosarcoma or fibrosarcoma.

3. Paget's disease.

4. Deposition of hemosiderin.

Reference

Manaster BJ, Doyle AJ: Giant cell tumors of bone. Radiol Clin North Am 31:299-323, 1993.

Comments

A GCT is a tumor that can demonstrate benign and malignant features and is sometimes referred to as a quasimalignant lesion. The pathologic and radiologic findings do not reflect the potential behavior of a lesion; therefore, it is difficult to predict which lesions are likely to be malignant. The incidence of malignancy has been estimated to be about 20%. Most GCTs present in the third or fourth decade of life, and 75% are discovered between the ages of 20 and 40 years. Although there is no sexual predilection for this tumor, the malignant form is three times more likely to occur in men. Typical presenting symptoms include pain and local swelling or diminished range of motion of a joint. Pathologic fractures occur in 10% of patients. The classic location is about the knee, composing more than 60% of all cases. The radiographic appearance of a GCT is an osteolytic, eccentrically located lesion in the metaphysis of the bone. In adults, it frequently extends to the articular surface of the bone, but in children the physis may impede the growth of the lesion into the epiphysis. Cortical thinning and mild expansion may be evident, and the margin of the lesion is often poorly demarcated. Magnetic resonance images may depict a sharper demarcation owing to the deposition of hemosiderin at the periphery of the tumor. The rate of recurrence after initial resection is estimated to be 40% to 60%.

Kienböck's Disease

1. Kienböck's disease.

2. Yes, collapse can be avoided with early diagnosis.

3. Most experts believe there is a relationship.

4. Computed tomography is preferred for acute trauma.

References

Gelberman RH, Bauman TD, Menon J, et al: The vascularity of the lunate bone and Kienböck's disease. J Hand Surg 5:272-278, 1980.

Lichtman DM, Alexander AH, Mack GR, Gunther SF: Kienböck's disease—update on silicone replacement arthroplasty. J Hand Surg Am 7:343-347, 1983.

Comments

Isolated lunate fractures are uncommon; however, this carpal bone is susceptible to Kienböck's disease—avascular necrosis of the lunate. The loss of the blood supply to the lunate has been attributed to primary fracture, repetitive trauma that causes microfractures, and traumatic injury to the ligaments that carry blood supply to the lunate. There is a statistical association among patients with an ulnar minus variant. The diagnosis is based on radiographic observations. Initially the lunate may appear normal, but with time the bone becomes increasingly sclerotic. This is followed by eventual loss of height, fragmentation, and subsequent collapse. Magnetic resonance imaging is useful in diagnosing the disease process earlier in patients with central wrist pain because marrow edema can be identified before sclerosis occurs.

Lichtman and colleagues devised a staging classification that identifies four different stages. In stage I, the radiographs are normal but magnetic resonance imaging may show areas of altered signal intensity or subchondral fracture. In stage II, the density of the bone increases. In stage III, the subchondral bone collapses. Two subtypes exist in stage III. In stage IIIA, there is lunate collapse by normal scaphoid rotation. In stage IIIB, the scaphoid rotation is fixed, and there may be advanced capitate collapse. In stage IV, arthritic changes develop throughout the carpus.

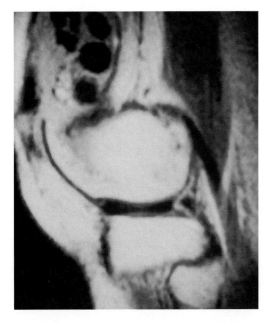

1. What causes the formation of intra-articular bodies in idiopathic synovial chondromatosis?

2. How do the intra-articular bodies ossify?

3. What percentage of patients with synovial chondromatosis do not have calcified or ossified intra-articular bodies? What is a helpful radiographic finding that differentiates this process from pigmented villonodular synovitis (PVNS)?

4. On magnetic resonance imaging (MRI), what differentiates chondromatosis from PVNS?

Idiopathic Synovial (Osteo)chondromatosis

1. Synovial metaplasia.

2. By endochondral ossification.

3. Twenty-five percent. Synovial chondromatosis rarely has an effusion, whereas PVNS commonly has a dense effusion.

4. In PVNS, one sees an effusion and hemosiderin deposition, and the nodular synovial masses show peripheral high signal intensity on T2W images. In chondromatosis, the cartilage nodules nearly always show a rim of low signal intensity on T2W images.

Reference

Kransdorf MJ, Meis JM: Extraskeletal osseous and cartilaginous tumors of the extremities. Radiographics 13:853–886, 1993.

Comments

Idiopathic synovial chondromatosis represents a synovial metaplasia of unknown etiology that is characterized by the formation of numerous cartilaginous nodules that project from the synovium into the joint. When the pedicle breaks, these nodules become detached into the joint cavity. Intra-articular nodules may resorb, enlarge, remain purely cartilaginous, or become calcified or ossified. When the nodules ossify, they do so by endochondral ossification, and the disease is more appropriately referred to as osteochondromatosis. The disease is monoarticular and affects young and middle-aged adults. Males are twice as affected as females. Clinically, a patient may relate a history of joint pain and limited range of motion lasting for several years. The most common joints involved are the knee, hip, elbow, and shoulder. The characteristic radiographic finding is numerous, small, calcified or ossified densities within the joint space. MRI usually reveals additional cartilaginous bodies that are not evident radiographically. These intra-articular nodules vary slightly in size but seldom exceed more than 2 to 3 cm in diameter. Pressure-erosive changes may develop in the intracapsular cortex, and mechanical effects of intra-articular bodies promote secondary osteoarthritic changes in the articular cartilage. Effusions, periarticular osteoporosis, and marginal erosions are not part of the radiographic spectrum. The differential diagnosis is quite limited and occasionally includes osteoarthritis, osteochondrosis dissecans, early neuropathic arthropathy, and PVNS.

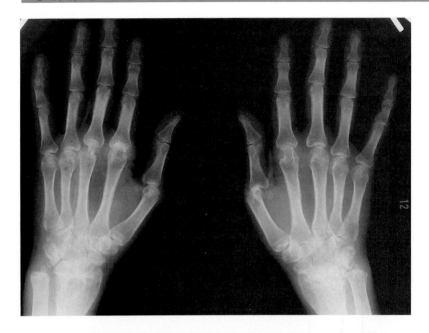

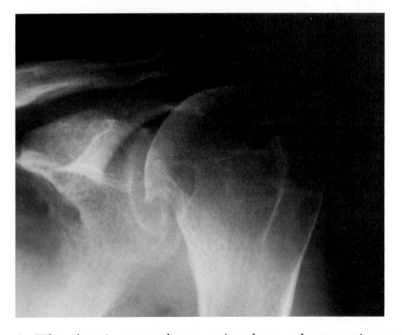

1. What does it mean when a patient has a robust-reactive type of rheumatoid arthritis (RA)?

2. What other disease processes manifest rheumatoid nodules?

3. What conditions can produce marked asymmetrical skeletal involvement in patients with RA?

4. What is Felty's syndrome?

Rheumatoid Arthritis

1. RA manifested by the presence of large radiolucent cysts found in patients who maintained a high level of activity during active disease.

2. Rheumatic fever, collagen-vascular diseases, sarcoidosis, Weber-Christian disease, gout, xanthomatosis, and infection.

3. Unilateral neurologic deficits, such as hemiparalysis or marked asymmetrical muscular weakness, that protect the ipsilateral side from the effects of RA.

4. RA, splenomegaly, and leukopenia.

Reference

Britton CA, Wasko MC: Rheumatoid arthritis. Semin Roentgenol 31:198–207, 1996.

Comments

The earliest pathologic abnormality of RA is acute synovitis, which is associated with synovial congestion and edema that cause hypertrophy and villous transformation of the synovium. Villous hypertrophy forms papillary fronds measuring 1 to 2 mm, and this may be evident on magnetic resonance imaging. The irregularity of the synovial tissue is most prominent at the edges of the articular cartilage. Pannus and toxic debris in the synovial fluid cause cartilaginous and osseous destruction. Histologically, cellular infiltration occurring diffusely or in small nodular aggregates, called Allison-Ghormley nodules, may be evident in the superficial portion of the synovium.

The characteristic radiographic features of RA include soft-tissue swelling, periarticular osteoporosis, early joint space narrowing, articular erosions, and marginal erosions caused by the extension of pannus into synovial pockets that expose regions that do not contain a protective cartilaginous layer (bare areas). In the shoulder, the anatomic neck demarcates the margin of the joint. An important observation in this patient is the lack of reactive changes about the erosions, because bony proliferation is not a part of the disease process. Although symmetry is the hallmark of RA, several exceptions are notable. Early in the disease process, involvement may be monoarticular or pauciarticular in 5% to 20% of patients. Stroke or other neurologic conditions that affect only one side of the body can cause asymmetrical joint involvement. And remember, in larger joints, involvement is occasionally asymmetrical as well.

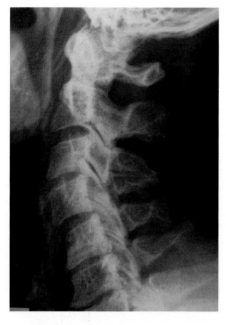

1. What is the major observation in this patient?
2. Name the joints that can encroach on the cervical canal if degenerated.
3. When patients with congenital stenosis develop spondylosis, what should be kept in mind?
4. In flexion and extension cervical spine radiographs, how much "listhesis" is considered normal?

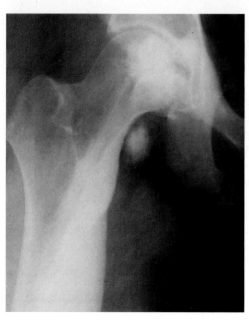
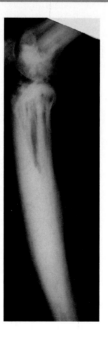

1. What is a sclerotome?
2. Name two lesions that are associated with melorheostosis of the axial skeleton.
3. How does this disorder progress radiographically?
4. What is osteopathia striata (Voorhoeve's disease)?

Congenital Spinal Stenosis

1. Diffuse congenital spinal stenosis.

2. Disk, apophyseal joint, and uncovertebral joint.

3. They become more vulnerable to cord injury because spondylosis further compromises a canal that is already too small.

4. Two millimeters or less.

Reference

Pavlov H, Torg JS, Robie B, Jahre C: Cervical spinal stenosis: Determination with vertebral body ratio method. Radiology 164:771–775, 1987.

Comments

Congenital spinal stenosis of the cervical spine is an important radiographic finding. Frequently, patients with a narrow canal present after trauma with transient sensory and motor symptoms in the arms, the legs, or all four extremities. Sensory changes may include numbness, burning, tingling, and paresthesia. Motor symptoms may include weakness and paralysis. When the injury is relatively minor, the neurologic symptoms are transient and may last for durations ranging from a few seconds to several minutes.

When the injury is more severe and involves significant axial loading, hyperextension, or hyperflexion, the symptoms may be permanent. The caliber of the cervical canal can be assessed by two methods on a lateral radiograph. In one method, the canal is measured from the posterior cortex of the vertebral body to the spinolaminar line. Symptoms of cord compression occur when the measurement is less than 10 mm. This technique does not correct for magnification, rotation, or variability in body size. A more useful technique is called the Pavlov ratio. In this method, the sagittal diameter of the spinal canal is divided by the sagittal diameter of the corresponding vertebral body. A ratio of 0.8 or less is considered significant and highly suggestive of congenital cervical spine stenosis.

Melorheostosis

1. Skeletal zones supplied by individual spinal sensory nerves.

2. Fibrolipomatous lesions and arteriovenous malformations.

3. Begins as linear hyperostosis, becomes uniform cortical thickening on one side of a bone, and progresses from one end of the bone to the center.

4. Dense linear striations in the metaphyses of bones.

Reference

Yu JS, Resnick D, Vaughan L, et al: Melorheostosis with an ossified soft tissue mass: MR features. Skeletal Radiol 24:367–370, 1995.

Comments

Melorheostosis, a rare, noninheritable, mesodermal disorder of unknown etiology, usually involves one bone or several bones distributed along the axis of a limb or along the distribution of a nerve. The hallmark of this process is progressive hyperostosis of bone. Melorheostosis is usually recognized in infancy and progresses during childhood and adult life. Chronic progressive pain in an affected limb is typical, and joint stiffness and decreased range of motion contribute to atrophy and weakness of the surrounding musculature. Para-articular soft-tissue ossification is rare but may be seen in more severely affected persons. Associated soft-tissue abnormalities include joint contractures, fibrosis and edema of the subcutaneous tissue, and varices. Pathologically, the sclerotic bone is composed of a mixture of immature and mature bone. Interlacing osteoid and thickened trabeculae eventually obliterate the haversian system. Fibrous tissue can be seen within the marrow spaces surrounding areas of new bone proliferation. Dense linear hyperostosis resembling "flowing candle wax" is the radiographic hallmark of this disease. The hyperostosis may advance to the joint margin or even protrude into the joint. Thickening of the cortex and adjacent underlying trabeculae is best demonstrated on computed tomography, whereas soft-tissue involvement is best depicted on magnetic resonance imaging. In this case, the findings are so characteristic that there is really no differential diagnosis.

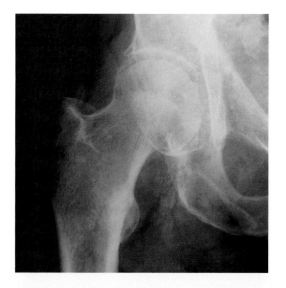
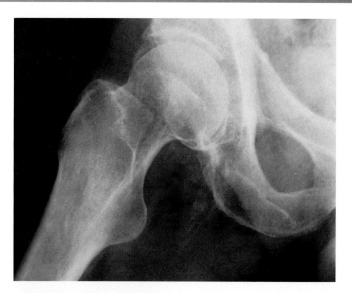
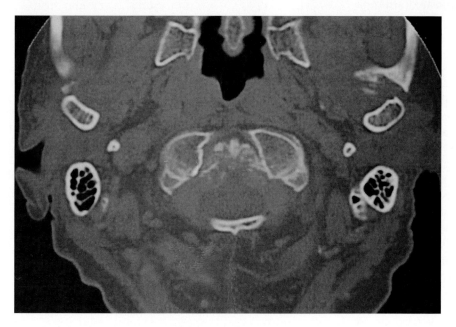

1. What is the etiology of the calcifications?

2. In tendons, can you differentiate hydroxyapatite from calcium pyrophosphate dihydrate (CPPD) crystal deposition?

3. Where is pyrophosphate arthropathy commonly detected?

4. Describe "rapidly progressive osteoarthritis."

CPPD Arthropathy and Enthesopathy

1. Deposition of calcium crystals.

2. Hydroxyapatite tends to be chunky and dense or cloudlike, whereas CPPD tends to appear thin and linear.

3. Knee, wrist, and second and third metacarpophalangeal joints.

4. Condition (usually in the hip) characterized by rapid development of degenerative changes depicted by extensive subchondral bone collapse and fragmentation, eburnation, joint space loss, and joint disorganization that often mimics neuroarthropathy. It is a misnomer because it represents a form of pyrophosphate arthropathy, not osteoarthritis.

Reference

Rubenstein J, Pritzke KPH: Crystal-associated arthropathies. AJR Am J Roentgenol 152:685-695, 1989.

Comments

The most important observation in this patient is chondrocalcinosis. Calcium is present in the hyaline cartilage and fibrocartilage of the labrum. Note also the extensive soft-tissue calcification in the region of the hip occurring at the enthesis of numerous tendons, including the insertion of the gluteal muscles (greater trochanter), the iliopsoas muscle (lesser trochanter), and the common tendon of the hamstring muscles (ischium). In the atlantoaxial junction of the cervical spine, chondrocalcinosis involves the syndesmo-odontoid region and the transverse ligament. CPPD crystals can accumulate in articular cartilage, synovium, capsule, tendons, and ligaments. When accumulation occurs in fibrocartilaginous tissues, such as the menisci of the knee, the triangular fibrocartilage of the wrist, the labrum of the hip, and the annular ligaments of the spine, it tends to appear thick, shaggy, and irregular. Synovial calcifications are often cloudlike, whereas capsular calcifications tend to be either linear or irregular. In the articular hyaline cartilage, calcifications appear thin and parallel the contour of the bony articular surface. Tendinous and ligamentous calcifications have a characteristic appearance of thin, linear, radiodense strands that often extend for a considerable distance from the bone.

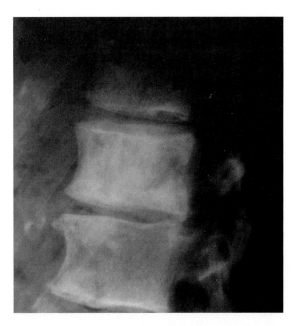 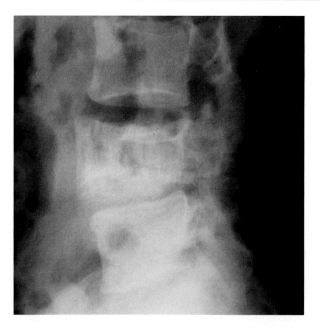

1. These two patients have the same condition. What is the diagnosis, and what percentage of patients presents with monostotic disease?
2. What are some findings that exclude the possibility of metastasis?
3. List several reasons why this patient could develop a neurologic complication.
4. What can happen if this condition affects the base of the skull? Why?

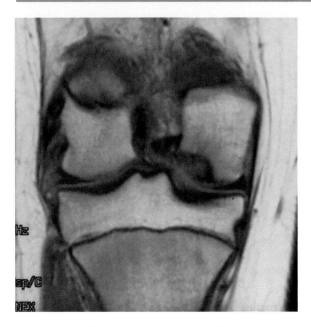

1. What is the diagnosis, and is this a common location?
2. What percentage of cases are bilateral?
3. Although the etiology of this lesion is unknown, how many patients reveal a history of trauma?
4. On magnetic resonance imaging, what is the most specific finding that is indicative of fragment instability?

Vertebral Paget's Disease

1. Paget's disease of the vertebral body. Ten to thirty-five percent.

2. Enlargement of the vertebral body, squaring of the anterior cortex, and involvement of the spinous process.

3. Vertebral body collapse, narrowing of the spinal canal owing to bone enlargement, stenosis of the neural foramina when there is involvement of the posterior elements, vascular steal syndrome from increased vascularity of pagetic bone, and mechanical interference with spinal cord blood supply.

4. Basilar invagination. The bone is relatively soft and allows the skull to settle.

Reference

Mirra JM, Brien EW, Tehranzadeh J: Paget's disease of bone: Review with emphasis on radiologic features, part II. Skeletal Radiol 24:173-184, 1995.

Comments

If you weren't careful on this case, you may have been tempted to embark on an "ivory vertebra" differential diagnosis. But in both patients, there is enlargement of the vertebral body, allowing you to safely render a diagnosis of Paget's disease. In the spine, involvement may be monostotic or polyostotic. The thickened cortex produces a classic "picture frame" appearance. Coarsening of the vertical trabeculation, along with the cortical changes, contributes to an increased density of the vertebral body. The lumbar spine and sacrum are the most common sites of involvement in the vertebral column. The cause of this disease is unknown. It is most common in middle-aged people and affects twice as many men as women. Paget's disease is characterized by osteoclastic activity in the lytic phase and osteoblastic activity in the reparative phase. Occasionally, collapse of the vertebral body occurs during the active phase of the disease, mimicking a neoplastic process. Progression of the disease to its quiescent phase produces the characteristic features depicted by this patient. Histologically, the lesions are characterized by fibrosis and marked vascularity. The haversian canals are abnormally enlarged, resulting in poor distinction between cortical and medullary bone.

Osteochondritis Dissecans

1. Osteochondritis dissecans. Yes, 80% of lesions occur in the medial femoral condyle, but the lateral femoral condyle, patella, and trochlea of the femur are uncommon sites.

2. Twenty-five percent are bilateral.

3. Nearly one half of patients.

4. Imbibition of joint fluid between the fragment and the rest of the femur. This finding correlates with fissuring of the articular cartilage.

Reference

Helgason JW, Chandnani VP, Yu JS: MR arthrography: A review of current technique and applications. AJR Am J Roentgenol 168:1473-1480, 1997.

Comments

Osteochondritis dissecans refers to a condition characterized by the development of a devascularized fragment of bone, usually in the non–weight-bearing surface of the medial femoral condyle. Radiographically, the lesion has a well-demarcated rim of sclerosis, which surrounds the abnormal marrow and extends to the articular cortex. Osteochondritis dissecans affects males two to three times more frequently than it affects females, and most patients present in adolescence (mean age of 15 years). The size of the osteochondral lesion and the thickness of the surrounding sclerotic rim are helpful when trying to stage a lesion. In stage I, a lesion measures approximately 1 to 3 cm in diameter, and the articular cartilage overlying the defect is intact. In stage II, the articular cartilage demonstrates a cleft or fissuring that extends to the cortex, but there is no indication of loosening of the fragment. In stage III, there is partial detachment of the osteochondral defect with a large cleft extending into the subchondral bone. In stage IV, the fragment is loose within the crater. Some investigators identify a fifth type in which there is a loose body and an empty crater. Magnetic resonance arthrography is the most accurate technique for establishing the stability of a lesion. Conventional T2W images may depict high signal intensity surrounding the osteochondral fragment, but it may be difficult to differentiate granulation tissue from free fluid. The formation of cysts deep to the lesion is associated with instability of the fragment, as is fluid imbibition between the fragment and the rest of the condyle.

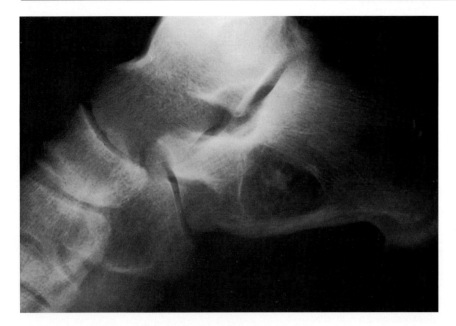

1. What entities would you consider?

2. Why is lipoid tissue bright in signal intensity on T1W magnetic resonance images?

3. How would you differentiate a calcaneal pseudocyst from a simple bone cyst or a lipoma?

4. What do you call a lipoma with increased vascularity? Is it malignant?

Intraosseous Lipoma

1. Intraosseous lipoma, simple bone cyst, and normal trabecular variation (pseudocyst).

2. Short T1 relaxation time.

3. A calcaneal pseudocyst is generally less prominent and less well defined than the other two kinds of lesions. It also tends to become more conspicuous with osteopenia.

4. An angiolipoma. No, but it can be infiltrative and invade locally and recur after excision.

Reference

Yu JS, Vitellas K: The calcaneus: Applications of MR imaging. Foot Ankle Int 17:771–780, 1996.

Comments

An intraosseous lipoma may be detected in patients of all ages. Histologically, this neoplasm is identical to an extraosseous lipoma; it is composed of mature adipose cells that are separated into lobules by fibrovascular septation. Two thirds of patients present with localized pain, which varies in duration. The most common location for this tumor is in the long bones of the lower extremity, with nearly 50% of cases involving the femur, tibia, and fibula. The calcaneus is the most common tarsal bone involved, accounting for 15% of all cases of intraosseous lipomas. A typical lesion appears well marginated, radiolucent, and surrounded by a thin rim of sclerosis. Lobulations are common at the margins of the lesion. In the calcaneus, it depicts a triangular configuration, typically residing between the major trabeculations of the bone, sharing a similar location with simple cysts. A central nidus of dystrophic calcification is common, which is nearly pathognomonic for this neoplasm. Unequivocal diagnosis is readily provided by T1W magnetic resonance images. The high signal intensity of the lipoma is demarcated from the fat in the bone marrow by a low signal intensity rim. Fat saturation is a nice technique for confirmation of tumor histology.

Fair Game

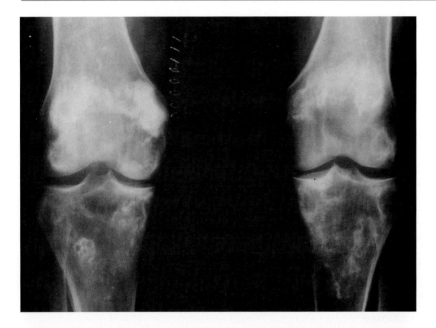

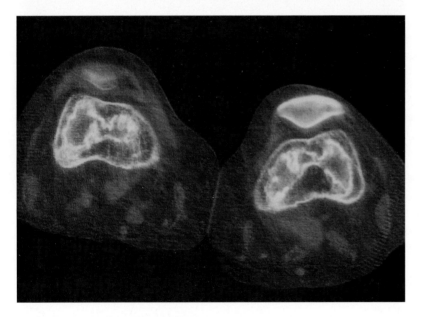

1. What is your differential diagnosis?

2. What is Gaucher's cell?

3. In pancreatitis, what causes bone infarctions? What is the subsequent effect of this process in the joints?

4. What causes the rim of sclerosis around an infarction?

Multifocal Steroid-Induced Osteonecrosis

1. Corticosteroid administration, hyperlipidemia, polycythemia, alcoholism, collagen vascular disease, hemoglobinopathies, Gaucher's disease, caisson disease, pancreatitis, and hyperuricemia.

2. Large cells (diameter 20 to 80 μm) in the reticuloendothelial system that contain cerebrosides in patients with Gaucher's disease.

3. Fat necrosis of the bone marrow. Polyarthritis associated with pain, swelling, tenderness, warmth, and effusion.

4. Mesenchymal cells that differentiate into osteoblasts, which synthesize new bone to encase the dead trabeculation.

References

Cruess RL: Steroid-induced avascular necrosis of the head of the humerus. Natural history and management. J Bone Joint Surg Br 58:313–317, 1976.

Fast A, Alon M, Weiss S, Zer-Aviv FR: Avascular necrosis of bone following short-term dexamethasone therapy for brain edema. Case report. J Neurosurg 61:983–985, 1984.

Comments

The association of osteonecrosis of bone and corticosteroid administration is important and is likely related to total intake of the substance. The maximum daily dose may be the most important factor, although no known safe dosage exists. A short-term, high-dose regimen is more likely to cause an infarction than are lower-dose regimens of longer duration. The cause-and-effect relationship remains unclear, although there are several hypotheses. A widely accepted theory suggests that corticosteroid induces adipose metamorphosis in the liver and hyperlipidemia. This leads to fat embolization and vascular occlusion in the bone. Another theory suggests that corticosteroid administration produces a hypercoagulable state of blood, which is associated with vasculitis. Yet another theory suggests that corticosteroids induce osteoporotic trabecular fractures, which compress the subchondral vascularity.

Patients present with pain and a limited range of motion in the joint nearest the infarction. Typically, the metaphysis and diaphysis of distal femur and proximal tibia are involved. The ischemic process may extend to the subchondral region of the epiphysis, ultimately causing articular collapse.

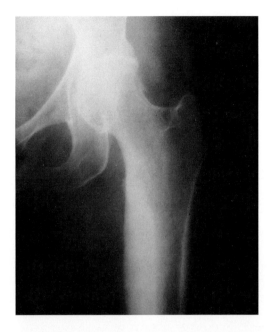
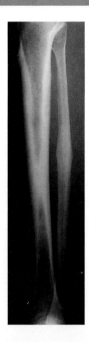
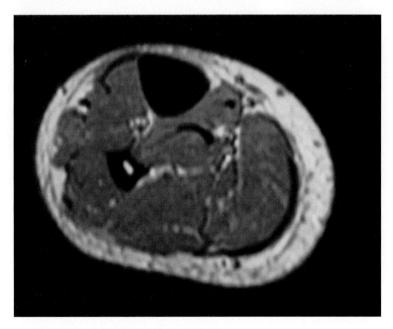

1. What is your differential diagnosis?

2. How do patients with Engelmann's disease present?

3. How would you differentiate Engelmann's disease from van Buchem's syndrome? Is there any other way to differentiate?

4. If only one bone were involved, what would you consider?

Engelmann's Disease

1. Consider the age of the patient: for children, Engelmann's disease, osteopetrosis, infantile cortical hyperostosis, and vitamin A poisoning; for adults, van Buchem's syndrome, hyperphosphatasemia, melorheostosis, Erdheim-Chester disease, Ribbing's disease.

2. Delayed walking with a wide-based gait in infancy (may be confused with muscular dystrophy).

3. Age: Engelmann's disease—young, van Buchem's syndrome—middle aged. Also, distribution: van Buchem's syndrome affects the bones of the hands, feet, pelvis, and ribs.

4. In this case, I think I would favor chronic infection.

Reference

Greenspan A: Sclerosing bone dysplasias—a target-site approach. Skeletal Radiol 20:561–583, 1991.

Comments

Engelmann's disease, or progressive diaphyseal dysplasia, is a bone dysplasia characterized by progressive formation of new bone along the cortices of tubular bones. The spectrum of proliferative changes ranges from very mild to severe. Symmetrical involvement of the long tubular bones, particularly the femur, tibia, humerus, and bones of the forearm, is common. The clinical manifestations of Engelmann's disease also cover a spectrum from asymptomatic to severe pain, muscle atrophy, weakness, and malnutrition. The usual age of onset is between ages 4 and 12 years. The characteristic radiographic finding is cortical thickening along the midshaft of a long tubular bone, involving both the periosteal and the endosteal surfaces. This proliferation of bone produces fusiform thickening of the diaphysis of the bone while simultaneously narrowing the medullary cavity. The resulting undertubulation causes an abrupt transition from the abnormal diaphysis to the uninvolved metaphysis. Small tubular bones of the hands and feet are infrequently affected, and the axial skeleton is rarely involved, except for the base of the skull. Ribbing's disease probably represents an adult form of Engelmann's disease. There is a familial incidence, and patients present during adolescence or young adulthood. The radiographic findings are nearly identical to those for Engelmann's disease.

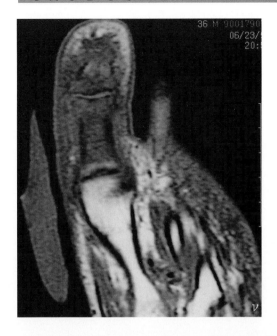

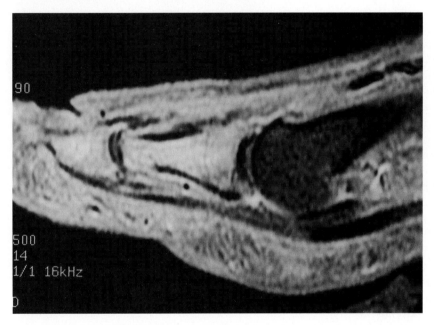

1. What is the differential diagnosis?

2. In the foot, how many plantar compartments are there, and why is it important to inspect them in an infection of the foot?

3. What causes an infected bone to appear dark on T1W and bright on T2W magnetic resonance images?

4. What causes enhancement of an infected bone after intravenous administration of gadolinium? Does this enhancement discriminate between edematous marrow and osteomyelitis?

Diabetic Osteomyelitis

1. Osteomyelitis of the proximal and distal phalanx of the great toe.

2. Three main compartments—medial, intermediate, and lateral. An infection may be contained by the intermuscular septa and spread proximally.

3. An alteration in the ratio of free water to bound water that prolongs the T1 and T2 tissue relaxation times.

4. Hyperemia. No.

Reference

Craig JG, Amin MB, Wu K, et al: Osteomyelitis of the diabetic foot: MR imaging—pathologic correlation. Radiology 203:849–855, 1997.

Comments

Osteomyelitis implies an infection of bone and marrow and is most commonly caused by bacterial agents, although fungi, parasites, and viruses can also infect the bone and marrow. There are three routes (hematogenous spread, direct extension, and direct implantation) that cause infection in the bone. Direct extension from an adjacent soft-tissue infection is the most common cause of osteomyelitis in a diabetic patient. In the hands and feet, skin ulceration is an important observation and requires close vigilance for an underlying infection. Furthermore, once the hands or feet become infected, the infection can spread through numerous structures and compartments, including the tendons, fascial planes, muscles, bones, and lymphatics. Infection caused by direct inoculation of the bone from a penetrating injury may be problematic because it may be associated with an unusual organism such as *Pseudomonas aeruginosa*. The radiographic features of osteomyelitis include osseous destruction, focal bone lysis, sclerosis, and periostitis, in addition to surrounding soft-tissue swelling or ulceration. Magnetic resonance imaging is useful for early detection of osteomyelitis because it allows direct inspection of the marrow. The use of gadolinium improves delineation of soft-tissue inflammatory masses but does not distinguish osteomyelitis from edema. It is therefore important to identify concomitant abnormalities such as an abscess, sinus tract, or skin ulceration.

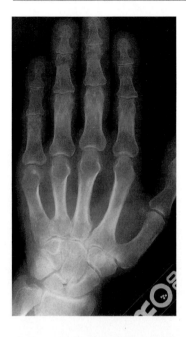

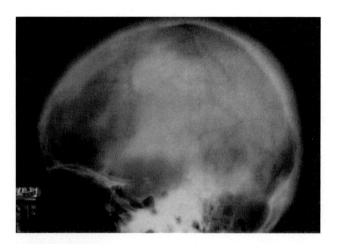

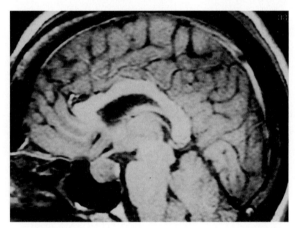

1. Identify the disease and its cause in this patient.
2. What is the sesamoid index?
3. List some expected abnormalities in the vertebral column.
4. What disease can mimic the radiographic and clinical findings evident in this patient?

Acromegaly

1. Acromegaly caused by a pituitary adenoma.

2. It is defined as the diameter of the medial sesamoid of the first metacarpophalangeal joint multiplied by the greatest perpendicular measurement (film performed at a 36-inch focus-film distance). Acromegaly is present when this value exceeds 40 in men and 33 in women.

3. Diffuse idiopathic skeletal hyperostosis–like condition, posterior scalloping, increased intervertebral height, elongation and widening of the vertebral bodies.

4. Pachydermoperiostosis.

Reference

Lang EK, Bessler WT: The roentgenologic features of acromegaly. AJR Am J Roentgenol 86:321-328, 1961.

Comments

Acromegaly is a condition caused by excess growth hormone generated from either pituitary hyperplasia or an adenoma. The effects of hyperpituitarism are broad and affect numerous organ systems, but defining markers are generally notable in the skeleton. A typical patient presents in the third or fourth decade of life and has a characteristic appearance: tall with prominent facial features (macrognathia, frontal bossing from enlarged frontal sinuses), poor dental occlusion, prominence of the tongue, and a spadelike hand with broad, separated fingers. Clinical complaints are of a rheumatic nature, including backache, peripheral arthropathy, compressive neuropathic symptoms such as carpal tunnel syndrome, and fatigue.

The key to the diagnosis in this patient is in the skull; the hand radiograph helps identify the effect of the pituitary adenoma. The sella turcica is enlarged, and there is erosion of a portion of the posterior wall. The cranial vault is thickened, and there is mild enlargement of the frontal sinuses. The magnetic resonance image demonstrates masslike enlargement of the pituitary gland. The close-up view of the fingers shows soft-tissue prominence and enlargement of the tuft of the terminal phalanx. Enlargement of the base of this bone is not prominent in this patient, but pronounced widening may produce a pseudoforamen.

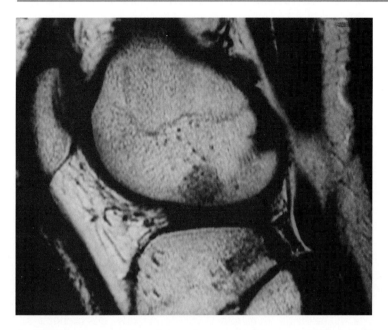 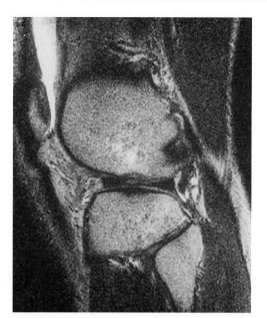

1. These two patients have the same diagnosis. What is the diagnosis?
2. What is identified histologically in the areas of altered bone marrow signal intensity?
3. Can this edema pattern occur with a partial tear of the anterior cruciate ligament (ACL)?
4. What are some radiographic signs that indicate an injury to the ACL?

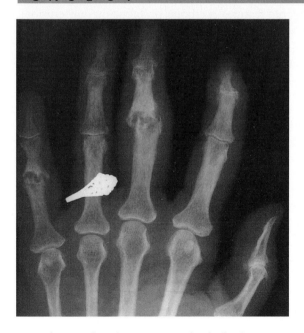

1. What is the diagnosis? Which findings are most characteristic of this arthropathy?
2. If only one joint was involved, what conditions would you have to consider in the differential diagnosis?
3. What is Cronkhite-Canada syndrome, and why would you consider this entity?
4. Does this patient have a risk of developing rheumatoid arthritis?

Rotary Contusion Pattern (ACL Tear)

1. Complete ACL tear.

2. Trabecular microfractures, hemorrhage, and interstitial edema.

3. For practical purposes, no.

4. Segond fracture, deep lateral notch sign, and avulsion of the anterior tibial eminence.

Reference

Yu JS, Cook PA: Magnetic resonance imaging (MRI) of the knee: A pattern approach for evaluating bone marrow edema. Crit Rev Diagn Imaging 37:261–303, 1996.

Comments

In the setting of acute trauma to the knee, bone marrow edema visualized on magnetic resonance images in the lateral femoral condyle and posterolateral tibia is nearly pathognomonic of a complete ACL tear. This contusion pattern occurs when the femur externally rotates on a fixed tibia. This mechanism of injury produces rotary subluxation of the femur while simultaneously displacing the tibia anteriorly. When the ACL ruptures, there is impaction of the articular surface of the lateral femoral condyle against the posterolateral aspect of the tibia, which produces the characteristic bone contusions. There are several other osseous abnormalities that, when visualized, should prompt close inspection of the ACL. They include a condylopatellar sulcus deeper than 1.5 mm produced by an osteochondral impaction of the lateral femoral condyle (deep lateral notch sign), a chip fracture of the posterolateral cortex of the proximal tibia created by shearing forces during subluxation of the femur, an avulsion of the anterior tibia at the attachment of the ACL, and an avulsion of the lateral tibial cortex at the attachment of the lateral capsular ligament (Segond fracture).

Erosive Osteoarthritis

1. Erosive osteoarthritis. Central erosions and soft-tissue swelling indicating an inflammatory process.

2. Erosive osteoarthritis, psoriatic arthritis, adult Still's disease, and septic arthropathy.

3. Gastrointestinal polyposis, hyperpigmentation of the skin, and nail atrophy. A variant of erosive osteoarthritis may be seen as a feature of this syndrome.

4. Yes, 15% develop full-blown features of rheumatoid arthritis.

Reference

Belhorn LH, Hess EV: Erosive osteoarthritis. Semin Arthritis Rheum 22:298–306, 1993.

Comments

Erosive osteoarthritis is an inflammatory form of osteoarthritis that affects predominantly postmenopausal, middle-aged women. It combines certain clinical manifestations of synovial inflammatory disease and the radiographic manifestations of osteoarthritis. Involvement is often limited to the hands, and the proximal and distal interphalangeal joints constitute preferred target sites. Early in the disease, patients present with a nonspecific synovial inflammatory arthropathy manifested by painful, swollen, and erythematous joints. The key radiologic features are bone proliferation and erosions. The proliferative changes are typical of osteoarthritis, as is its distribution. The articular erosions that develop tend to be centrally located, creating large defects in the cortex and subchondral bone. Osteophytes that develop at the margins of the joint result in a characteristic "gull wing" appearance, although this finding may be seen in other arthritides. Ankylosis of the interphalangeal joint, not seen in noninflammatory osteoarthritis, can occur in the erosive form. Approximately 15% of patients with erosive osteoarthritis develop clinical, laboratory (elevated erythrocyte sedimentation rate and positive rheumatoid factor), and radiographic manifestations of rheumatoid arthritis. However, the exact relationship between these two conditions remains unclear.

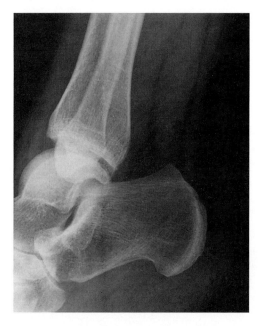

1. What is your diagnosis?

2. When do patients usually present, and with what symptoms?

3. What other common anomalous muscle may cross Kager's fat pad?

4. When patients present with exercise-induced claudication, what is the preferred treatment?

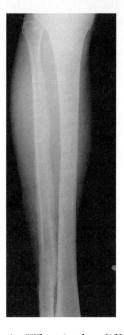 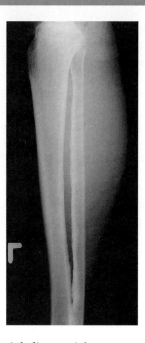

1. What is the differential diagnosis?

2. What clues do you look for if you suspect venous stasis?

3. In chronic pachydermoperiostosis, what happens to the peripheral blood flow, and why? And in secondary hypertrophic osteoarthropathy?

4. Can arterial insufficiency cause periosteal bone proliferation?

Accessory Soleus Muscle

1. Accessory soleus muscle.

2. Late adolescence or young adulthood. Patients present with a mass, soft-tissue swelling, or claudication.

3. Peroneus quadratus (quartus) muscle.

4. Fasciotomy.

Reference

Yu JS, Resnick D: MR imaging of the accessory soleus muscle. Skeletal Radiol 23:525–528, 1994.

Comments

This patient has an accessory soleus muscle. At the level of the tibiotalar joint, only two muscles should be visualized—the flexor hallucis longus and peroneus brevis muscles. Posterior to these muscles is a large fat pad, called Kager's fat pad, which has the appearance of a large triangular radiolucency with the Achilles tendon marking its posterior border and the calcaneus marking its inferior border. When a soft-tissue mass is detected in Kager's fat pad, one should consider the possibility of an anomalous muscle. An accessory soleus muscle is best depicted on magnetic resonance imaging. On sagittal images, it characteristically appears as a fusiform-shaped soft-tissue mass demonstrating T1 and T2 values identical to those of normal muscle. On transaxial images, the muscle appears as a sharply marginated, ovoid mass seen at the level of the tibiotalar joint. This muscle is enveloped by its own fascia, deriving its blood supply from the posterior tibial artery and innervation from the posterior tibial nerve. It arises from either the anterior surface of the soleus muscle or the soleal line of the tibia and fibula. It may insert into the Achilles tendon, the upper surface of the calcaneus, or the medial aspect of the calcaneus.

Periostitis of Vascular Insufficiency

1. Secondary hypertrophic osteoarthropathy, pachydermoperiostosis, venous stasis, thyroid acropachy, hypervitaminosis A.

2. Evidence of vascular disease such as soft-tissue swelling and ulcers and phleboliths.

3. Decreased, either from thickening of the arterial wall or from connective tissue overgrowth, which compresses small and medium-sized arteries. Increased.

4. Yes, in polyarteritis nodosa and other arteritides.

Reference

Resnick D, Niwayama G: Enostosis, hyperostosis, and periostitis. In Resnick D (ed): Diagnosis of Bone and Joint Disorders, 3rd ed. Philadelphia, WB Saunders, 1995, pp 4396–4466.

Comments

When assessing a patient with periosteal changes in the bone, several important considerations include skeletal distribution (e.g., upper or lower extremity, peripheral or proximal, hands), epiphyseal and metaphyseal involvement, pattern of periostitis (e.g., thin, thick, single layer, multiple layers), symptoms (pain), and systemic conditions (e.g., venous stasis, infection, pleural disease). An important observation in this case is identifying involvement of the cortex of the tibia, where the periostitis is quite subtle. This enables you to entertain a differential diagnosis of diffuse periostitis in contradistinction to periostitis involving only one bone. Another important observation is a large ulceration in the lateral aspect of the lower leg surrounded by soft-tissue swelling. The periosteal pattern is typical of venous stasis, with undulating new bone appearing in the diaphyses and metaphyses of the tibia and fibula but sparing the epiphyses. An important consideration to remember is that initially the periosteal new bone may be separated from the cortex, but it will later merge with it. A more nodular and irregular appearance probably indicates a superimposed soft-tissue infection.

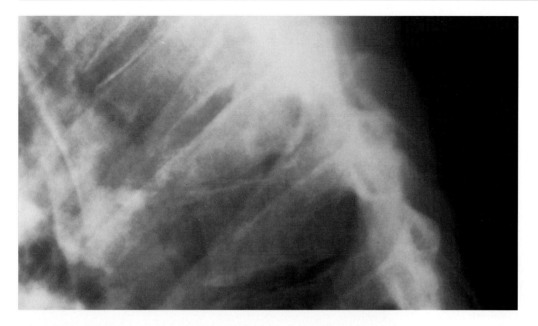

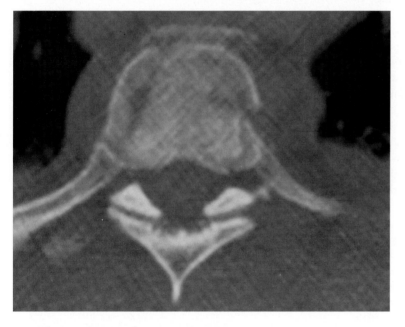

1. What is the mechanism of injury?
2. Is this considered a stable injury?
3. What finding would render a simple compression fracture unlikely?
4. How frequent are neurologic deficits with this fracture?

Burst Fracture (T5 Vertebra)

1. Axial loading.

2. No.

3. Retropulsion of the middle column.

4. About 50% of patients with an acute burst fracture suffer from a neurologic deficit. However, there is no direct relationship between the extent of spinal canal narrowing and the severity of the deficit.

Reference

Denis F: The three column spine and its significance in the classification of acute thoracolumbar spinal injuries. Spine 8:817–831, 1983.

Comments

Compressive axial loading of the vertebral body, which produces end-plate failure and vertebral body collapse, is the principal cause of burst fractures of the spine. The force of the axial load dictates the morphology of the fracture. When the axial force is small, a simple compression fracture is produced. As the force increases, vertical fractures develop throughout the body. Assessment of spinal stability can be achieved by applying the Denis three-column model of the spine. In this model, the spine is divided into three columns: the anterior column is composed of the anterior half of the vertebral body and disk, anterior annulus fibrosus, and anterior longitudinal ligament; the middle column is composed of the posterior vertebral body and disk, posterior annulus fibrosus, and posterior longitudinal ligament; and the posterior column is composed of the posterior osseous and ligamentous structures. Unstable fractures are defined as injuries in which two of the three columns are involved. Often, when the middle column is involved, the injury is unstable when caused by axial loading. As the axial load increases, there is displacement of the bone fragments and retropulsion into the spinal canal. Ultimately, when the axial force overwhelms the pedicle junction, the interpediculate distance may widen, causing significant disruption of the posterior elements.

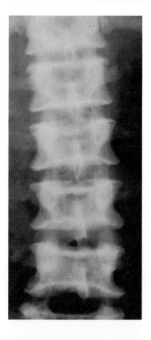 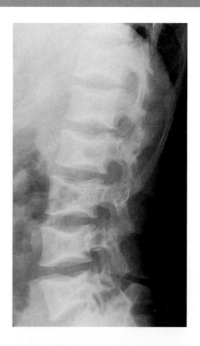

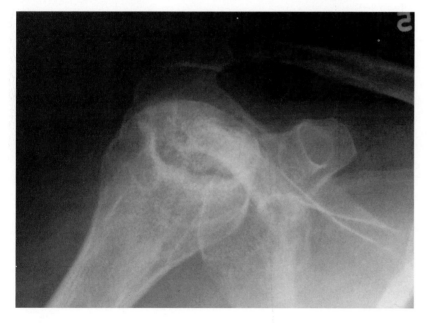

1. What is the diagnosis?
2. Describe hand-foot syndrome. Whom does it affect?
3. What is the most important determinant of disease severity?
4. Where do we see a "tramline" sign, and in whom?

Sickle Cell Disease

1. Sickle cell disease.

2. Acute dactylitis from ischemia. Black infants age 6 to 18 months (uncommon after age 6 years).

3. Oxygen tension.

4. Infarction in the cortex causes it to split apart. Older patients.

Reference

Crowley JJ, Sarnaik S: Imaging of sickle cell disease. Pediatr Radiol 29:646–661, 1999.

Comments

Sickle cell disease occurs primarily in black persons and in persons of a Mediterranean descent. It is an inherited disorder that is characterized by reversible sickling of the red blood cells. People who carry two genes for sickle hemoglobin (HbSS) have sickle cell anemia. People who have only one gene for sickle hemoglobin have sickle cell variants. Only a few of these variants have important clinical expressions. When HbS is found in combination with HbC or thalassemia, the process is referred to as sickle cell disease. Several factors influence the severity of the disease. Oxygen tension is the most important factor in patients with sickle cell disease because sickling begins when the oxygen tension drops below 40 mm Hg. Other important considerations include pH, blood viscosity, mechanical fragility of red blood cells, and percentage of HbS. Clinically, patients present with anemia caused by rapid destruction of the abnormal erythrocytes. The increased blood viscosity causes thrombosis and infarction in end vessels, which may present as dactylitis in infants.

Radiographically, there is coarsening of the osseous trabeculation and diminished bone density. The vertebral bodies demonstrate characteristic biconcave contours ("fish vertebrae") or central depressions that are the result of diminished bone growth induced by sludging of red blood cells. The bone-in-bone appearances in the long bones are created by infarctions. Hip and shoulder pain may indicate the presence of avascular necrosis.

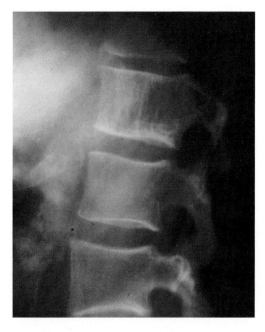 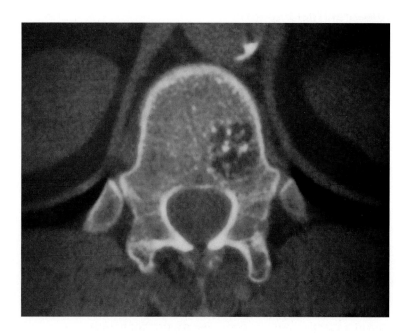

1. How common is this lesion?

2. The majority of patients who have this lesion are asymptomatic. But how might it cause symptoms?

3. Which cross-sectional imaging technique more reliably shows the reinforced trabeculation in the lesion, computed tomography (CT) or magnetic resonance imaging (MRI)?

4. Where do conventional hemangiomas occur? And compressive hemangiomas?

Vertebral Hemangioma

1. It is present in as much as 10% of the population.

2. By compression of the spinal cord, cauda equina, or nerve root if the lesion expands the posterior elements of the vertebra, and—rarely—by compression of the neural structures by extension of the hemangioma into the epidural space.

3. CT, overwhelmingly.

4. Conventional—thoracic and lumbar spine; compressive—more than 90% occur in thoracic spine.

Reference

Laredo JD, Reizine D, Bard M, Merland JJ: Vertebral hemangiomas: Radiologic evaluation. Radiology 161:183–189, 1986.

Comments

This is a straightforward case of a conventional hemangioma of a lumbar vertebral body. The majority of hemangiomas are incidental findings on x-rays, presenting as a solitary abnormality. It is the most common benign lesion of the spine and has a characteristic appearance. Hemangiomas are not true tumors because they consist of dilated blood vessels, which cause resorption of the bony trabeculation. The remaining compressive trabeculation thickens, yielding a classic "corduroy" appearance depicted on radiographs of the spine. On CT, the prominent vertical trabeculation is demonstrated as a polka-dot pattern inside a well-defined osteolytic area with a fatty stroma (attenuation <30 HU). On MRI, a heterogeneous pattern of increased signal intensity may be seen on both the T1W and the T2W images, reflecting the signal properties of the lipoid stroma. The cortex is generally intact, and there is no associated soft-tissue mass. A compressive vertebral hemangioma, which is more aggressive but much less common than a conventional hemangioma, frequently involves the entire vertebral body and extends to the neural arch. Owing to an angiomatous stroma, rather than to the fatty stroma of a conventional hemangioma, compressive vertebral hemangiomas may mimic a vascular neoplasm or metastasis. They have a higher attenuation value (>20 HU), and the signal intensity on T2W images can be very intense.

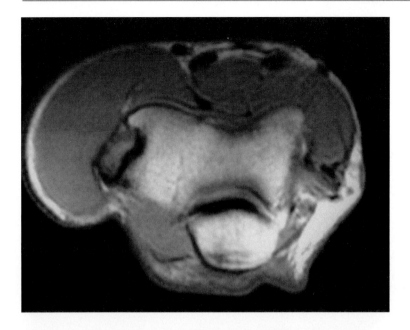

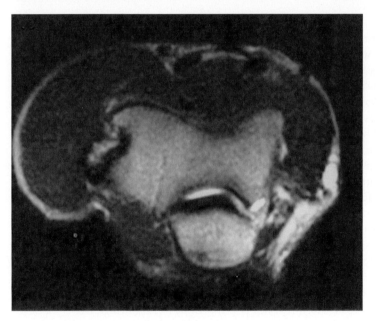

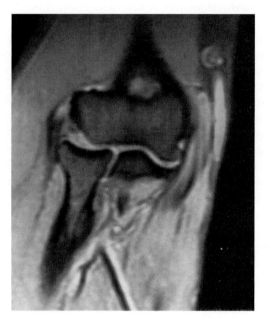

1. What does this patient have?
2. Is bone marrow edema in the humerus common in patients with this condition?
3. How is it treated?
4. In pediatric patients, what condition mimics medial epicondylitis?

Lateral Epicondylitis

1. Lateral epicondylitis.

2. Occasionally, but the term *epicondylitis* is a misnomer because the majority of patients suffer from tendinosis of the common forearm flexor and extensor tendons.

3. The majority of patients respond to conservative therapy consisting of rest, nonsteroidal anti-inflammatory drugs, and occasional immobilization. Longitudinal tenotomy and tendinous releases are reserved for those with recalcitrant conditions.

4. Avulsion of the medial epicondylar ossification center.

Reference

Martin CE, Schweitzer ME: MR imaging of epicondylitis. Skeletal Radiol 27:133–138, 1998.

Comments

The term *epicondylitis* refers to an overuse syndrome characterized by pain and tenderness over the epicondylar portions of the elbow caused by repetitive motion. Lateral epicondylitis is common in tennis players and is the result of repeated rotary forearm motion. Medial epicondylitis is common in baseball pitchers and is the result of forceful flexion of the elbow. The diagnosis of epicondylitis can be confirmed on magnetic resonance imaging in the acute phase of the disease. The magnetic resonance features of both overuse syndromes include thickening of the tendinous insertions; altered signal intensity in the tendon in both T1W and T2W images that correlates with areas of fibroangiomatous hyperplasia and hyaline degeneration (tendinosis); and, occasionally, edema in the adjacent bone marrow. Acute avulsive injuries may be accompanied by interstitial edema (characterized by marked high signal intensity on T2W images) in the tendon, and these signal changes are more pronounced than are those that occur in tendinosis. Periosteal reaction may also be noted, particularly on inversion recovery images, which does not ordinarily occur in tendinosis. Chronic changes may be detected radiographically and consist of dystrophic calcification at the enthesis of the tendon and cortical irregularity at the humeral epicondyles.

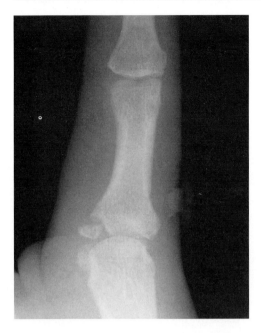

1. What injury does this patient have?

2. How is this injury produced?

3. Why have we moved away from stress radiography for confirmation of ulnar collateral ligament (UCL) injuries?

4. What is the treatment of choice for nondisplaced injuries like the one shown by this patient? Why is this treatment appropriate?

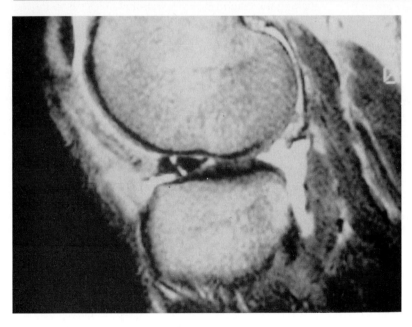

1. What is the diagnosis?

2. Why is this injury a relative emergency?

3. What other conditions should you consider when you see an "absent meniscus" sign?

4. Describe the double posterior cruciate ligament (PCL) sign.

Gamekeeper's Thumb

1. Avulsion of the base of the proximal phalanx of the thumb at the attachment of the UCL.

2. Violent abduction of the thumb, which either disrupts the ulnar collateral ligament or causes an avulsion of its osseous insertion.

3. Potential for creating Stener's lesions.

4. Conservative therapy with immobilization. The UCL is a capsular ligament, and nonsurgical management is adequate for healing, as with medial collateral ligament injuries of the knee.

Reference

Spaeth HJ, Abrams RA, Bock GW, et al: Gamekeeper thumb: Differentiation of nondisplaced and displaced tears of the ulnar collateral ligament with MR imaging. Radiology 188:553–556, 1993.

Comments

An injury to the UCL of the metacarpophalangeal joint of the thumb is termed *gamekeeper's thumb.* It accounts for approximately 6% of all skiing injuries but is also a frequent injury in athletic activities such as football, wrestling, baseball, and hockey. In the past, the diagnosis was based on clinical examination and stress radiography. More recently, magnetic resonance imaging has been advocated for evaluation of UCL injuries. When the UCL ruptures, the torn end may become displaced superficially to the adductor pollicis aponeurosis. This complex, called *Stener's lesion,* may interfere with healing because the interposed aponeurosis prevents apposition of the ligament to the bone. In this situation, surgery has been advocated as the treatment of choice because instability may persist if the injury is left untreated. When the UCL avulses from the base of the proximal phalanx of the thumb, the relative position of the bone fragment may allow differentiation between a nondisplaced tear and Stener's lesion. If radiographic evaluation fails to demonstrate an osseous avulsion, then further evaluation with magnetic resonance imaging to ensure that the ligament is not displaced is recommended. In the past, injuries of the UCL were confirmed with stress radiography, but it is now realized that a nondisplaced tear may be easily displaced with this maneuver and will then require surgical repair.

Buckethandle Tear (Lateral Meniscus)

1. Buckethandle tear of the lateral meniscus with a flipped fragment.

2. Patients should be treated expeditiously because these tears may cause joint locking.

3. Prior meniscectomy, large meniscal tear, congenital hypoplasia or aplasia, and severe degeneration.

4. Buckethandle tear of the medial meniscus with displaced intercondylar fragment that mimics the appearance of the PCL on sagittal magnetic resonance images.

Reference

Magee TH, Hinson GW: MRI of meniscal bucket-handle tears. Skeletal Radiol 27:495–499, 1998.

Comments

Buckethandle tears of the knee have been reported to occur in 9% to 24% of patients with a meniscal tear. It is the most common cause of a displaced meniscal injury and may be due to a longitudinal, vertical, or oblique tear. It often involves the entire length of the meniscus, although isolated involvement of the anterior or posterior horn can occur. A meniscal fragment can be displaced into the intercondylar notch or the anterior compartment.

Magnetic resonance imaging is the best noninvasive technique for detecting buckethandle tears. A key to making the diagnosis on the coronal images is to inspect the intercondylar region closely for abnormal structures and the menisci for a cleft that divides the peripheral fragment (bucket) from the displaced fragment (handle). Several important signs that are indicative of a buckethandle tear have been identified on the sagittal images. The double PCL sign indicates that a displaced intercondylar fragment lies inferior to the PCL, paralleling the orientation of this ligament. This finding has been reported only with medial meniscal tears. The "flipped meniscus" sign refers to a buckethandle tear that has tears at two points. When the peripheral fragment displaces anteriorly, it becomes juxtaposed to the anterior horn, giving the appearance that the meniscal horn has a "piggyback" companion. This finding frequently accompanies an "absent meniscus" sign.

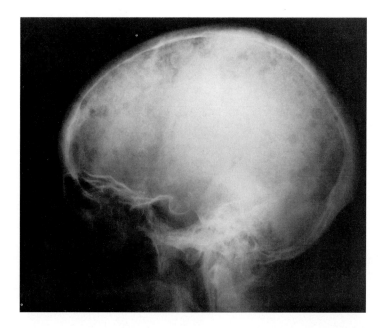

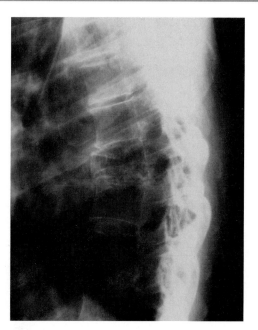

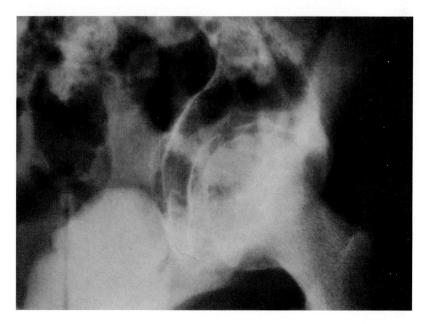

1. What are the finding in the spine and the differential diagnosis?
2. Why is the serum calcium level elevated?
3. What is a Bence Jones protein? Who has them?
4. Define the POEMS syndrome. Why is this disease peculiar?

Multiple Myeloma

1. Pathologic fracture of the T8 vertebral body. Osteoporosis, trauma, multiple myeloma, metastasis, benign lesion such as hemangioma.

2. It is mobilized from the bones.

3. The light polypeptide chain of an immunoglobulin. Patients with multiple myeloma, lymphomas, metastatic bone tumors, idiopathic hemolytic disease, and essential cryoglobulinemia.

4. Polyneuropathy, organomegaly (hepatosplenomegaly), endocrine dysfunction, M-protein, and skin abnormalities. The myelomatous lesions are sclerotic.

Reference

Meszaros WT: The many facets of multiple myeloma. Semin Roentgenol 9:219–228, 1974.

Comments

Multiple myeloma is a primary malignancy of bone that originates in the hematopoietic bone marrow, causing its replacement by proliferating cells that resemble plasma cells. It is this replacement of bone that is depicted as osteopenia. It is the most common primary bone malignancy involving the osseous elements. Ninety-eight percent of people who are affected are older than 40 years, and this neoplasm is considered rare in persons younger than 30 years. There is a 2:1 male predilection. The disease usually is widespread, but occasionally a solitary lesion may occur, referred to as a *plasmacytoma*. Early in the disease, symptoms may be insidious. Constitutional symptoms such as fever and anemia are common. Disease progression elicits bone pain, particularly in the spine, where pathologic fractures are common and cord compression can cause paraplegia. Computed tomography or magnetic resonance imaging best evaluates this complication. Radiographic changes in the bone are evident in 65% to 75% of patients and include osteopenia, focal lytic lesions, and pathologic fractures. Lytic lesions are characteristically small and well defined and create a "punched out" appearance. Occasionally, they may have a bubbly, expansile appearance. The key to the diagnosis in this case is the multiplicity of sites involved. By overlapping the differential lists for lesions that cause a bubbly appearance and lesions that cause pathologic fractures in osteopenic vertebral bodies, you should be able to narrow your differential diagnosis to metastasis and multiple myeloma. Then all you need to do is wait for the result of the serum electrophoresis.

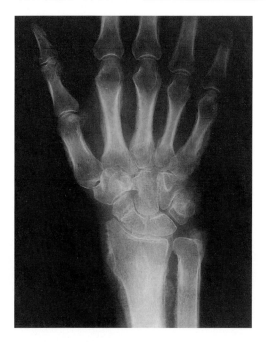 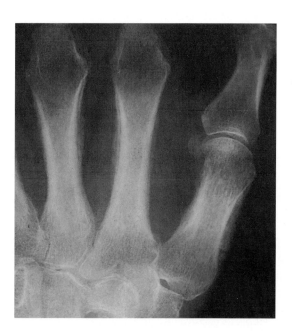

1. What would you expect to see on a bone scan? Is a bone scan more sensitive than radiographs?

2. Is this a painful condition?

3. What articular manifestations may occur in this patient?

4. Is there an association with acro-osteolysis?

Secondary Hypertrophic Osteoarthropathy

1. "Parallel track" sign (tracer uptake along the cortical margins of the metaphysis and diaphysis of the tubular bones of the extremities). Yes.

2. Yes. In fact, pain differentiates hypertrophic osteoarthropathy (HOA) from thyroid acropachy, which is painless.

3. Periarticular osteoporosis, joint effusions, and soft-tissue swelling mimicking rheumatoid arthritis.

4. There can be focal areas of distal tuft resorption that mimic acro-osteolysis.

References

Pineda CJ, Fonseca C, Martinez-Lavin M: The spectrum of soft tissue and skeletal abnormalities of hypertrophic osteoarthropathy. J Rheumatol 17:626–632, 1990.

Pineda CJ, Martinez-Lavin M, Goobar JE, et al: Periostitis in hypertrophic osteoarthropathy: Relationship to disease duration. AJR Am J Roentgenol 148:773–778, 1987.

Comments

Secondary HOA, also known as *hypertrophic pulmonary osteoarthropathy,* is a chronic proliferative bone disorder characterized by painful periostitis of long tubular bones, clubbing of the fingers and toes, and synovitis. The periostitis causes a relatively acute, deep-seated pain in the extremities, often described as a severe burning, and the adjacent skin may be swollen and warm. In contradistinction to primary HOA (pachydermoperiostosis), a form that is often hereditary but is occasionally idiopathic, secondary HOA is associated with an underlying neoplastic, infectious, or inflammatory process, which accounts for 95% of all cases of HOA. About 10% to 25% of patients with bronchogenic carcinoma develop HOA, as do as many as 50% of patients with pleural mesothelioma.

Radiographically, periosteal new bone may be evident in the diaphysis of the tibia and fibula, radius and ulna, femur, humerus, metacarpals and metatarsals, and phalanges. It is a bilateral process as seen in this patient's right-hand radiograph and in the close-up view of the left hand. As the disease progresses, the metaphyseal regions of these bones become involved. The differential diagnosis includes primary HOA, thyroid acropachy, and venous stasis. In thyroid acropachy, the periostitis is asymptomatic and occurs principally in the small bones of the hands and feet. It does not involve the long tubular bones. Other clinical findings, such as exophthalmos and pretibial myxedema, are generally present as well. Periosteal reaction in venous stasis tends to occur in the lower extremities.

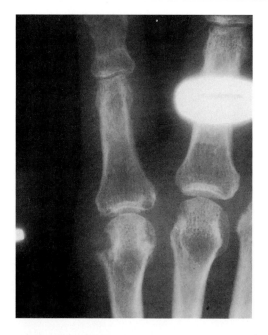

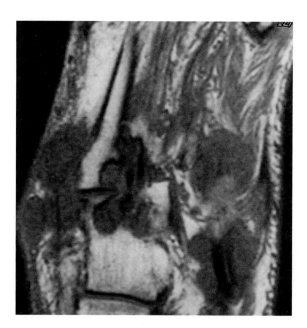

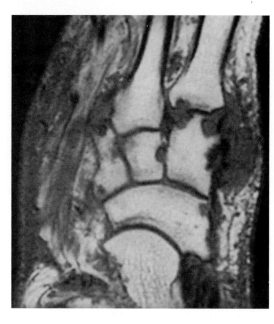

1. Is there a genetic predisposition to the primary form of this disease?

2. What is a typical time interval from onset of symptoms to radiographically detectable changes in the joints?

3. On magnetic resonance imaging, what causes bone marrow edema in a patient with this disease?

4. What characterizes Lesch-Nyhan syndrome? Who is affected?

Gout

1. Yes, autosomal dominant with weak penetrance in females (90% of patients affected are male).

2. Many years (average 7 to 12 years).

3. Intraosseous migration of monosodium urate crystals and synovitis.

4. Mental retardation, self-mutilation, choreoathetosis, hyperuricemia, and uric acid nephrolithiasis. Males (X-linked recessive).

Reference

Yu JS, Chung C, Recht M, et al: MR imaging of tophaceous gout. AJR Am J Roentgenol 168:523–527, 1997.

Comments

Gout is a condition caused by the deposition of urate monohydrate crystals in tissues. Gout can be divided into an idiopathic form and those forms that are secondary to other disorders. The idiopathic form is characterized by an overproduction of uric acid owing to abnormal renal excretion of urate, caused by a deficiency of the enzyme phosphoribosyltransferase. There are numerous causes of secondary gout. In some diseases, the increased production of uric acid is caused by an excessive breakdown of nucleoproteins (polycythemia vera, myelofibrosis, leukemia, multiple myeloma, anemias, psoriasis, and glycogen storage disease), whereas in others, it is caused by renal failure.

The key to this case is not to be overwhelmed by the findings. Because many arthropathies coexist, you need to ask yourself these questions: "Is the same process affecting all the joints?" and, if so, "Which joint best characterizes the disease?" The fifth metacarpophalangeal joint is fairly characteristic of this disease process. Notice that a rim of sclerosis surrounds all the marginal erosions and that the erosions in the ulnar aspect of the fifth metacarpal head and about the fifth tarsometatarsal joint result in prominent, "overhanging" edges. Despite numerous erosions, the joint space is relatively well maintained, and the bone density is nearly normal. On magnetic resonance imaging, gout can sometime mimic a neoplastic process, because it can provoke a significant periosteal reaction and bone marrow edema. Destruction of the bone and the presence of juxta-articular masses (which do enhance) can appear ominous to the wearied observer. The key to interpreting gout on magnetic resonance imaging is to identify a lesion that is low in signal intensity on both T1W and T2W images. There are not many "bad things" that have low signal intensity on T2W images. Once you have performed this task, you can resume your search for features that are typical of gout.

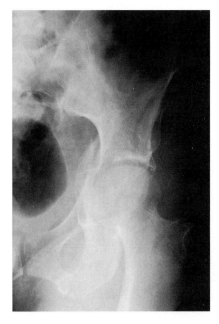

1. Are acetabular fractures common? What is the most common type?
2. How can you differentiate a column fracture from a transverse fracture of the acetabulum on computed tomography (CT)?
3. Radiographically, what are several important osseous landmarks that enable you to assess the acetabulum?
4. Central dislocations frequently accompany what type of acetabular fracture?

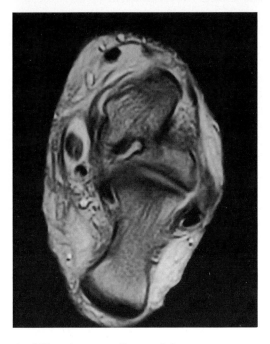

1. What is your diagnosis?
2. Where are the insertions of the posterior tibial (PT) tendon?
3. What is a potential consequence of a complete rupture of the PT tendon? Who is at risk for a rupture?
4. What features differentiate an os tibiale externum from a true accessory navicular?

Acetabular Fractures

1. Yes, these injuries constitute 25% of all pelvic fractures. Acetabular wall fractures.

2. Column fracture is oriented in the coronal plane of the pelvis, whereas a transverse fracture is oriented in the sagittal plane.

3. The iliopectineal and ilioischial lines identify the columns, and the anterior and posterior rim lines identify the acetabular margins.

4. Transverse, T-shaped, and transverse-posterior wall fractures.

Reference

Yu JS: Hip and femur trauma. Semin Musculoskeletal Radiol 4:205–220, 2000.

Comments

Fractures of the acetabulum occur as a result of high-energy trauma and are frequently complex because of comminution. The displacement of multiple fragments may result in incongruity of the articular surface and ultimate development of posttraumatic osteoarthritis. The Judet-Letournel classification has been widely recognized as a useful surgical classification. Fractures of the acetabulum are divided into five simple fracture types and five associated fracture types representing a combination of different simple fracture types. The simple fracture types are posterior acetabular wall, posterior column, anterior acetabular wall, anterior column, and transverse acetabular fractures. The five associated fracture types are transverse and posterior acetabular wall, T-shaped, anterior column and posterior hemitransverse, posterior column and posterior acetabular wall, and both column fractures.

CT is advocated for evaluating acetabular fractures. The advantage of CT over conventional radiography is unimpeded visualization of complex fractures, allowing more accurate assessment of the size, relationship, and degree of displacement of fracture fragments, incongruity at fracture lines, and disruption of the acetabular column. Column and transverse fractures have characteristic imaging patterns on CT. Anterior and posterior column fractures are oriented in a medial-to-lateral orientation (coronal plane). These fractures extend into the obturator foramen. Transverse fractures bisect the innominate bone and are oriented in the anterior-to-posterior direction (sagittal plane).

Posterior Tibial Tendon Tear

1. Tear of the PT tendon.

2. Navicular, medial and intermediate cuneiform, and base of the 2–4 metatarsals.

3. Can lead to progressive pes planus deformity and weakened inversion. Women in fifth or sixth decades of life.

4. Os tibiale externum is small (2 to 6 mm), round, separate from the navicular, and encompassed by the PT tendon; an accessory navicular is in continuity with the navicular by a synchondrosis, is triangular in shape, and may be the site of insertion of the PT tendon.

Reference

Rosenberg Z, Cheung Y, Jahss M, et al: Rupture of the posterior tibial tendon: CT and MR imaging with surgical correlation. Radiology 169:229–235, 1988.

Comments

The PT tendon is the most frequently injured tendon in the medial aspect of the foot. Patients present with pain, local tenderness, and swelling. On magnetic resonance imaging, the PT tendon has an ovoid configuration. Its normal diameter is two to three times the size of the adjacent flexor digitorum longus tendon. There are three patterns of rupture of the PT tendon. A type 1 tear is characterized by longitudinal splitting of the tendon, producing a thickened morphology owing to hemorrhage and fibrous tissue. The tendon may be four to five times its normal size and may depict heterogeneous signal intensity changes. Type 2 tears are more severe tears resulting in thinning or attenuation (atrophy) of the tendon. In type 3 tears, there is a complete tendon rupture with retraction and gap between the proximal and distal fibers. The gap usually fills with either fluid or hemorrhage. A significant number of patients with symptoms related to the PT tendon are afflicted with tendinosis. Fusiform thickening of the tendon associated with degenerative signal intensity changes on T1 and T2W images is a characteristic magnetic resonance feature of this noninflammatory disorder. In these patients, the pathologic process is often insidious, and symptoms may mimic arch instability.

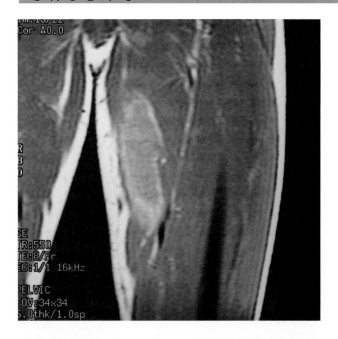

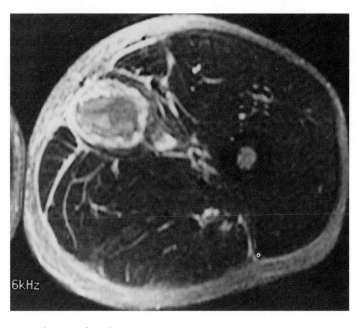

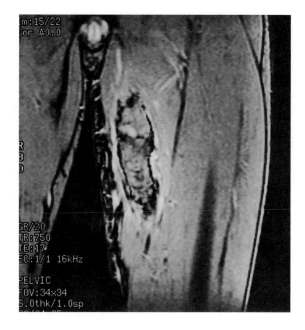

1. What is the diagnosis?

2. High signal intensity on T1W images is indicative of what?

3. What magnetic resonance sequence enhances the conspicuity of hemosiderin? Is the effect related to magnetic field strength?

4. Does intracellular deoxyhemoglobin exhibit a paramagnetic effect? What is its effect?

Intramuscular Hematoma

1. Gastrocnemius tear and formation of an intramuscular hematoma.

2. Extracellular methemoglobin seen in a subacute hematoma.

3. Gradient-recalled echo sequence. Yes.

4. Yes. It lowers signal intensity on T2W images.

References

Gomori JM, Grossman RI, Goldberg HI, et al: Intracranial hematomas: Imaging by high-field MR. Radiology 157:87-93, 1985.

Gomori JM, Grossman RI, Yu-Ip C, et al: NMR relaxation times of blood: Dependence on field strength, oxidation state, and cell integrity. J Comput Assist Tomogr 11:684-690, 1987.

Comments

The extravasation of blood into the soft tissues occurs either as an intraparenchymal hemorrhage (not confined to a definite space and freely dissecting around muscle fascicles and fascial layers) or as a hematoma (confined blood cavity). The appearance of an intramuscular hematoma depends on its size, location, active bleeding, and length of existence. Differing oxygen tension, absorption of extravasated blood, and degradation of hemoglobin are factors that alter the appearance of a hematoma, and the effect of these factors is initially more pronounced at the periphery of a hematoma than at its center. Hemoglobin is broken down sequentially into both paramagnetic and nonparamagnetic substances. High signal intensity on T1W images is caused by the strong paramagnetic effect of methemoglobin, while deoxyhemoglobin exhibits its paramagnetic effect on T2W images. As such, a hematoma may have a complex and evolving appearance on magnetic resonance imaging.

In general, an acute hematoma is isointense with muscle on T1W images and hypointense on T2W (deoxyhemoglobin). As the hematoma evolves, the hematoma depicts higher signal intensity on T2W images and eventually on T1W images (methemoglobin). If it becomes a chronic seroma, it may exhibit low signal intensity on T1W images and high signal intensity on T2W images. A low signal intensity rim that becomes exaggerated on gradient-recalled echo images is related to the accumulation of hemosiderin. But remember that the hypointensity patterns of deoxyhemoglobin and hemosiderin are proportional to the square of the magnitude of the mean magnetic field, so their effects are more pronounced at a high field strength than at a low magnetic field strength.

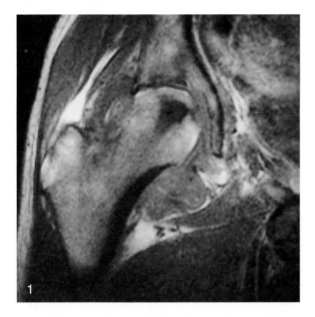 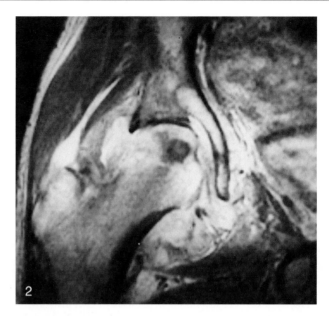

1. What is the most likely diagnosis? Is it benign or malignant?
2. Is matrix calcification a common finding?
3. On magnetic resonance imaging (MRI), is it common to identify peritumoral edema surrounding this lesion?
4. Histologically, are hemorrhagic cysts associated with this lesion? Would it affect the MRI appearance?

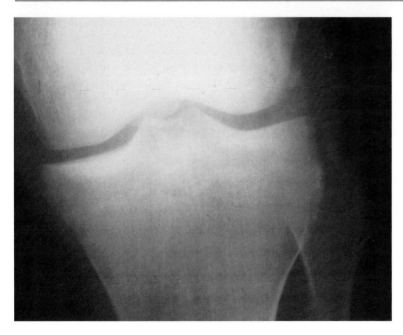

1. What is your diagnosis, and what does it imply?
2. What is the classic mechanism of injury?
3. If you had only the bone scan, what would you consider?
4. What injuries would you expect to find on a magnetic resonance imaging (MRI) examination?

Chondroblastoma

1. A chondroblastoma. Benign.

2. Yes, it may be seen in 30% to 50% of cases.

3. Identification of peritumoral edema is very common owing to the hypervascularity associated with this lesion.

4. Yes, they may even resemble an aneurysmal bone cyst in 10% of cases. Yes.

References

Oxtoby JW, Davies AM: MRI characteristics of chondroblastoma. Clin Radiol 51:22–26, 1996.

Weatherall PT, Maale GE, Mendelsohn DB, et al: Chondroblastoma: Classic and confusing appearance at MR imaging. Radiology 190:467–474, 1994.

Comments

Chondroblastoma is a benign tumor of bone characterized by chondroblasts and multinucleated giant cells. Nearly 90% of patients present between the ages of 5 and 25 years, and there is a twofold male predilection. The most common complaint is pain referring to a joint. Tenderness, swelling, decreased range of motion, numbness, muscle atrophy, and weakness may be discovered on physical inspection. The femur (33%), humerus (20%), and tibia (20%) are usual sites of involvement, although about 10% of chondroblastomas occur in the bones of the hands and feet, especially in the talus and calcaneus. The radiographic hallmark of this tumor is a well-defined osteolytic lesion that is centrally or eccentrically located within the epiphysis or apophysis of a bone. A thin sclerotic rim surrounds the lesion, separating it from the normal marrow. Calcifications may be evident in 30% to 50% of cases. Periostitis is notable in one third of all cases. Aggressive features, such as joint invasion and extension into the adjacent soft tissue and bones, and marked enhancement are not uncommon. The differential diagnosis includes infection and eosinophilic granuloma, although these lesions have their epicenters in the metaphysis of the bone. A giant cell tumor generally occurs in the epiphysis of a bone but lacks matrix calcification or a sclerotic rim.

Segond Fracture

1. Segond fracture. An anterior cruciate ligament tear.

2. Rotational or twisting injury with external rotation of the femur on a fixed tibia.

3. Stress fracture, acute infarction, occult fracture.

4. Injuries to the anterior cruciate ligament (80% to 100%), medial collateral ligament (80% to 90%), meniscus (50%), and articular cartilage (25%).

References

Dietz GW, Wilcox DM, Montgomery JB: Segond tibial condyle fracture: Lateral capsular ligament avulsion. Radiology 159:467–469, 1986.

Goldman AB, Pavlov H, Rubenstein D: The Segond fracture of the proximal tibia: A small avulsion that reflects major ligamentous damage. AJR Am J Roentgenol 151:1163–1167, 1988.

Comments

This lesion was initially described in 1879, when Segond demonstrated that internal rotation of the tibia with the knee in flexion resulted in tension of the lateral joint capsule. When the tension exceeded the strength of the bone, a small avulsion fracture occurred in the lateral tibia about 4 mm distal to the lateral joint line. Radiographically, the abnormality ranges from a small vertical sliver of bone to a sizable bone fragment. The importance of this fracture is that it has a strong association with rupture of the anterior cruciate ligament. The Segond fracture can sometimes be mistaken for other injuries in the lateral aspect of the knee because this fracture is not apparent on lateral radiographs. Avulsion of the lateral collateral ligament may simulate a Segond fracture, but the bone fragment tends to be displaced more proximally and posteriorly than does the Segond fracture. You should look for a concomitant abnormality in the fibular head when you suspect this injury. Studies suggest that an iliotibial band avulsion may constitute a variation on the Segond injury.

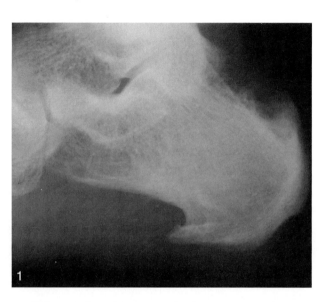
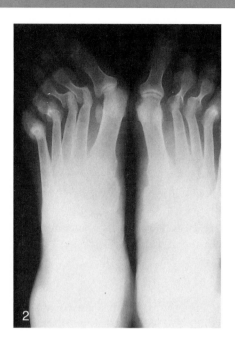

1. What is the classic triad of Reiter's syndrome?

2. There are two common mucocutaneous manifestations associated with Reiter's syndrome. Name them. How often can you see them?

3. Does Reiter's syndrome affect the heart?

4. Approximately how many patients with Reiter's syndrome have positive human leukocyte antigen (HLA)-B27?

Reiter's Syndrome

1. Arthritis, conjunctivitis, and urethritis.

2. Balanitis circinata sicca (inflammation of the glans penis) and keratoderma blennorrhagicum (hyperkeratosis and spongiform pustules). They occur in 50% of patients.

3. Yes, conduction abnormalities and aortic regurgitation can occur.

4. About 75%.

Reference

El-Khoury GY, Kathol MH, Brandser EA: Seronegative spondyloarthropathies. Radiol Clin North Am 34:343–357, 1996.

Comments

Reiter's syndrome is an arthropathy that affects males between the ages of 20 and 40 years, 4 weeks to 4 months after they recover from an infection of the bowel or lower genitourinary tract. The onset of arthritis is acute, characterized by pain, erythema, and warmth, and it affects several joints. There is a predilection for the joints of the lower extremity. The heel is one of the primary target sites of this seronegative arthropathy. Osseous proliferation begins as fluffy periostitis at the enthesis of the plantar aponeurosis and Achilles' tendon. Poorly defined erosions soon develop on these entheses, but this finding is nonspecific and is characteristic of all the seronegative arthropathies, including psoriatic arthritis and ankylosing spondylitis. Retrocalcaneal bursitis may produce erosions along the posterosuperior surface of the calcaneus, in a similar fashion to rheumatoid arthritis.

Edema, erythrocyte extravasation, and infiltration of neutrophils and lymphocytes characterize the synovial inflammation in the acute phase of Reiter's syndrome. When the synovitis is more chronic, there is villous hypertrophy and pannus formation. The metatarsophalangeal and interphalangeal joints of the foot are common target sites, demonstrating asymmetrical involvement with soft-tissue swelling and fluffy periostitis initially. As the disease progresses, characteristic findings include joint space narrowing, marginal erosions, and subluxation of the metatarsophalangeal joints. Sacroiliitis is a bilateral and asymmetrical process that eventually affects 40% to 60% of patients.

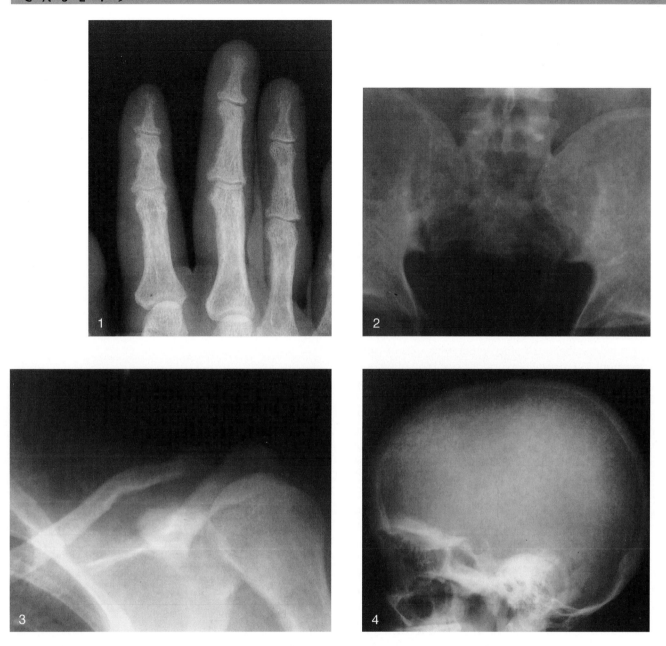

1. List the types of bone resorption characteristic of hyperparathyroidism. Which ones are shown?
2. Why is this not sacroiliitis?
3. The rugger-jersey spine is a manifestation of what type of bone resorption?
4. What is a brown tumor?

Bone Resorption in Hyperparathyroidism

1. Subperiosteal, endosteal, intracortical, subchondral, trabecular, and subligamentous. Subchondral (pelvis, distal clavicle), subperiosteal (phalanges), and trabecular (skull).

2. The joint space is not narrowed, and a thin rim of the cortex overlying the resorbed bone is evident.

3. Subchondral type.

4. Localized accumulations of fibrous tissue, giant cells, and osteoclasts, which replace the bone in patients with hyperparathyroidism.

Reference

Resnick D, Niwayama G: Parathyroid disorders and renal osteodystrophy. In Resnick D (ed): Diagnosis of Bone and Joint Disorders, 3rd ed. Philadelphia, WB Saunders, 1995, pp 2012–2075.

Comments

The radiologic hallmark of hyperparathyroidism is bone resorption. There are six types of bone resorption: subperiosteal, endosteal, intracortical, subchondral, trabecular, and subligamentous. The sacroiliac joints are a common location for subchondral resorption and may mimic the radiographic findings of sacroiliitis. The iliac side is more severely involved, and cartilage fibrillation and subchondral bone erosion are accompanied by reactive new bone formation. Radiographically, this produces ill-defined joint margins that may appear widened (actually pseudowidened because the cortices are not completely absent). Subchondral resorption is also common at the acromioclavicular and sternoclavicular joints and the discovertebral junctions. Trabecular resorption is a prevalent manifestation of advanced hyperparathyroidism and occurs in the medullary cavity throughout the skeleton. It is usually conspicuous in the skull because resorbed bone is replaced by connective tissue containing newly formed trabeculae, producing a loss of definition between the tables of the skull. It also results in the characteristic "salt and pepper" appearance shown in this patient.

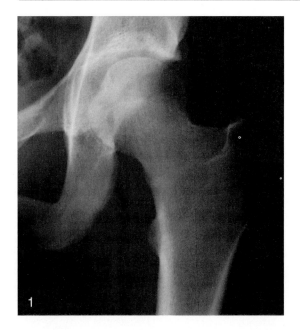

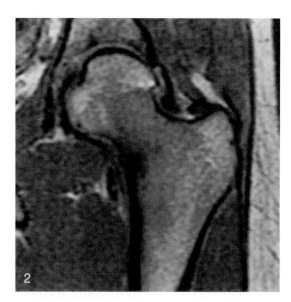

1. Define a fatigue fracture and an insufficiency fracture.

2. What is the most constant feature in the clinical history of patients with fatigue fractures?

3. What is the best imaging technique for evaluating longitudinal or vertical stress fractures of the femur?

4. What condition commonly presents with a tensile insufficiency fracture?

Femoral Neck Stress Fractures

1. Fatigue fracture is caused by abnormal stresses applied to normal bone, whereas an insufficiency fracture is caused by normal stresses on abnormal bone.

2. New onset or increased intensity of a particular strenuous and repetitive activity.

3. Computed tomography. The marrow edema pattern depicted on magnetic resonance imaging is confusing and may suggest a more ominous process.

4. Paget's disease.

Reference

Arendt EA, Griffiths HJ: The use of MR imaging in the assessment and clinical management of stress reactions of bone in high-performance athletes. Clin Sports Med 16:291–306, 1997.

Comments

Stress fractures of the femoral neck are more common than are fractures that occur in the diaphysis. Clinically, patients complain of hip pain that radiates to the knee, although point tenderness may be difficult to elicit on examination. Early diagnosis and treatment are essential because this type of stress fracture may proceed to become a complete fracture. Because the abnormality is often radiographically occult, magnetic resonance imaging has been shown to be particularly useful in identifying these fractures. T1W images provide the best contrast for depicting the low signal intensity fracture, whereas inversion recovery images provide the greatest sensitivity for marrow edema.

Femoral stress fractures are classified as either compressive or tensile. Compressive stress fractures occur at the base of the femoral neck, near the calcar femorale in the medial aspect of the bone. This type of stress fracture is by far more common than tensile stress fractures and are commonly seen in athletes. Occasionally, it is associated with focal fusiform thickening of the periosteum, caused by callus formation mimicking an osteoid osteoma. Compressive stress fractures do not usually displace and can be treated with simple non–weight bearing. Tensile stress fractures, on the other hand, tend to occur in older patients. The bone may have an underlying abnormality. A defect in the superior cortex of the femoral neck will progress to a complete fracture, with displacement in 50% of patients, if it is not treated appropriately. Once a fracture line is visible, internal fixation may be indicated.

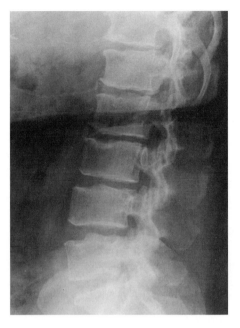

1. Whom does this disease affect?
2. What is the clinical significance of this diagnosis?
3. What is the pathogenesis?
4. Can this disease affect only the lumbar spine?

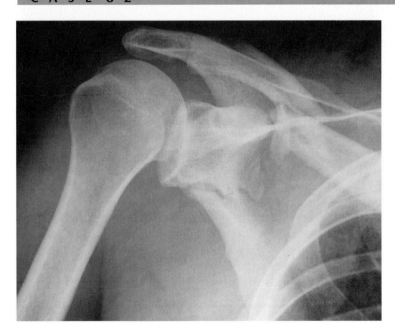

1. Identify the injuries.
2. How does this injury occur?
3. If this injury remains untreated, what eventually happens to the joint?
4. What are two common humeral fractures associated with this injury, and how frequently do they occur?

Scheuermann's Disease

1. Adolescents—young men more frequently than women—age 10 to 18 years.

2. Early degenerative disk disease and higher incidence of compression fractures.

3. Congenital defects in the anterior aspect of the end plates that allow herniation of the nucleus pulposus.

4. Yes, as many as 25% of cases may be seen in the lumbar spine only.

Reference

Resnick D: Osteochondroses. In Resnick D (ed): Diagnosis of Bone and Joint Disorders, 3rd ed. Philadelphia, WB Saunders, 1995, pp 3595–3600.

Comments

This disease is considered one of the osteochondroses, affecting the vertebral body epiphysis. A narrow, ring-like epiphysis forms along the superior and inferior margins of the vertebral body during the second decade of life. The disease is painful and affects children between the ages of 10 and 18 years. When they are affected with Scheuermann's disease, the epiphyseal plates lose their sharp outlines and become fragmented and sclerotic. The adjacent border of the vertebral body also becomes irregular as a result of a growth disturbance of the epiphysis, and this leads to a wedge-shaped deformity of the anterior vertebral body. Involvement of several bodies results in an exaggerated dorsal kyphosis, which may develop rapidly during the course of the disease. The lower thoracic and upper lumbar vertebrae are most frequently targeted. In some patients several vertebral bodies may be involved, whereas in others the entire spine may be affected.

After the disease heals, residual irregularities of the end plate may persist. Anterior wedging of the vertebral body and kyphotic curvature are permanent findings. Radiographically, Schmorl's nodes (protrusion of the nucleus pulposus into the end plate) are common at multiple levels as well as at deficient portions of the anterior epiphyseal plate, causing a notchlike defect in the anterior corner of the vertebral body. Narrowed disk spaces with calcifications are common.

Posterior Shoulder Dislocation

1. Posterior shoulder dislocation and scapular fracture.

2. As a result of indirect trauma, such as electrocution or seizure, but occasionally as a result of direct impact against the anterior shoulder or falling on an outstretched hand.

3. Development of pseudoarthrosis and glenohumeral instability.

4. Lesser tuberosity fracture (25%) and humeral head (10%).

References

Cisternino SJ, Rogers LF, Stufflebam BC, Kruglik GD: The trough line: A radiographic sign of posterior shoulder dislocation. AJR Am J Roentgenol 130:951–954, 1978.

Schwartz E, Warren RF, O'Brien SJ, Fronek J: Posterior shoulder instability. Orthop Clin North Am 18:409–419, 1987.

Comments

A posterior dislocation of the glenohumeral joint is one of the most commonly misdiagnosed injuries in trauma patients. About 50% of these injuries are missed on initial radiographic evaluation. Several factors contribute to the errors in diagnosis. An adequate study may be impossible to perform because the shoulder is locked in internal rotation. Clinically, important findings that are indicative of a dislocation may be masked by concomitant hematoma, muscle spasm, or associated fractures. A lesser tuberosity fracture of the proximal humerus should raise your suspicion for a potential posterior glenohumeral dislocation. There are three types of posterior shoulder dislocations; however, nearly all cases are the subacromial type. Posterior subglenoid and subspinous dislocations are rare. Important radiographic observations include the trough sign (a vertical compression fracture of the anterior humeral head), the rim sign (widening of the joint beyond 6 mm), the absent half-moon sign (loss of humeral head–glenoid rim overlap), Velpeau's sign (superior subluxation of the humeral head), and disruption of the scapulohumeral arch. Computed tomography should be performed when a posterior dislocation is suspected to search for a reverse Bankart lesion, tear of the posterior labrum, and stripping of the posterior periosteum.

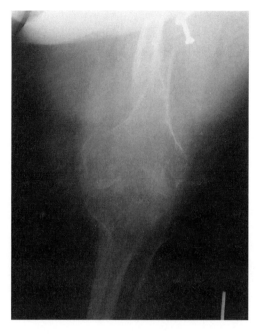

1. List the clinical manifestations of this disease.

2. Can patients with this disease have normal-appearing sclerae?

3. What radiographic observations may be identified in the skull of patients with this condition?

4. At what age does otosclerosis occur in affected patients?

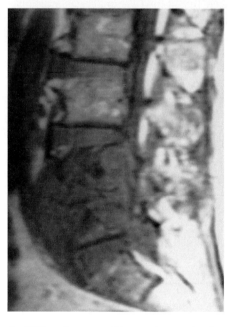 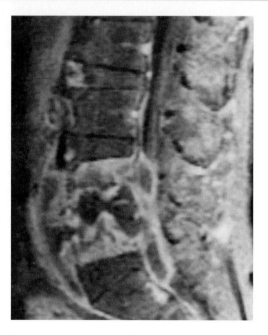

1. What is your diagnosis, and what findings support your diagnosis?

2. List three mechanisms by which the spine may become infected.

3. What is the classic magnetic resonance appearance of a pyogenic spondylitis? What is the most common organism cultured?

4. What is different about the spine in children that allows hematogenous seeding of the disk?

Osteogenesis Imperfecta

1. Skeletal fragility from osteoporosis, blue sclerae, dentinogenesis imperfecta, and premature otosclerosis.

2. Yes, in type 4 subtype.

3. Platybasia, basilar invagination, wormian bones, enlarged sinuses, and abnormal teeth.

4. Before age 40 years.

Reference

Silence D: Osteogenesis imperfecta: An expanding panorama of variants. Clin Orthop 159:11-25, 1981.

Comments

Osteogenesis imperfecta (OI) is an inherited disorder of connective tissue that affects the synthesis and quality of fibrillar collagen, producing a form of congenital osteoporosis. The incidence of OI is one in 20,000 to 60,000 births. There are two main forms: a congenital form (10%) and a tarda form that affects the majority of patients. Each form is further subdivided into two types. The congenital types, types 2 and 3, are severe and characterized by multiple fractures at birth. Both these subtypes are likely inherited as an autosomal recessive trait. The latent types, types 1 and 4, are inherited as an autosomal dominant trait. In these patients, the incidence of fractures varies, and only 20% of patients with these subtypes present with fractures at birth. In type 1 OI, the classic tarda form, the first fracture typically occurs in the second or third year of life. Radiographically, the classic findings include marked osteopenia and slender and overconstricted tubular bones. The cortices may appear either thinned or thickened. Deformities from previous fractures may be dominant findings, or bones may appear bowed secondary to microfractures. Excessive callus formation is a characteristic finding of the disease and may involve the entire length of the bone, although some fractures may heal with a pseudoarthrosis. Ligamentous laxity causes premature degenerative joint disease.

Tuberculous Spondylitis

1. Tuberculous spondylitis. Large epidural and paraspinal abscesses, subligamentous spread to L2-L3 and L3-L4 disks anteriorly, periostitis of L3, and peridural spread to S2 posteriorly.

2. Hematogenous source, direct implantation by way of the venous system (Batson's plexus), or direct extension from an adjacent infection.

3. Edema involving two contiguous vertebral bodies with a narrowed intervertebral disk. *Staphylococcus aureus.*

4. Persistent blood supply to the disk.

Reference

Bell GR, Stearns KL, Bonutti PM, Boumphrey FR: MRI diagnosis of tuberculous vertebral osteomyelitis. Spine 15:462-465, 1990.

Comments

This patient presented with characteristic findings of a tuberculous spondylitis (Pott's disease). Clinically, patients present with back pain, although localized tenderness and stiffness and a neurologic deficit also are common initial complaints. On magnetic resonance imaging, tuberculous spondylitis may appear identical to pyogenic spondylitis. Low signal intensity in the subchondral region of the end plate on T1W images, which becomes moderately bright on T2W images, is indicative of edematous infected marrow. The infection can erode the articular cortex and then penetrate into the disk, where the infection is free to spread to the adjacent vertebral body. Remember that tuberculous spondylitis has several notable differences from bacterial infections, because the posterior elements, disk, epidural space, and paraspinous soft tissues can also become primarily infected along with the vertebral body. The loss of cortical distinction in the anterior or posterior aspect of the vertebral body correlates with extension of the infection beneath the longitudinal ligaments, and this process is often expressed in the form of periostitis. The development of an acute, angular kyphosis (gibbus deformity) is strongly suggestive of tuberculosis. Tuberculosis may also directly infect the paraspinal soft tissues, creating large abscesses, particularly in the psoas muscles. The infection can extend via the longitudinal ligaments, paraspinal soft tissues, and muscles, producing skip lesions far removed from the initial source of infection. Another typical feature of tuberculosis is a "burrowing" abscess. These tubular tracts can also course for a long distance and perforate the internal organs of the peritoneal cavity or communicate to the skin through a sinus.

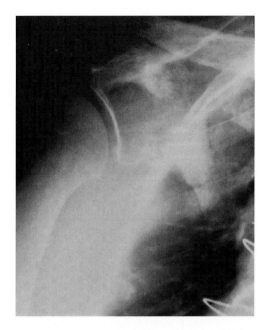
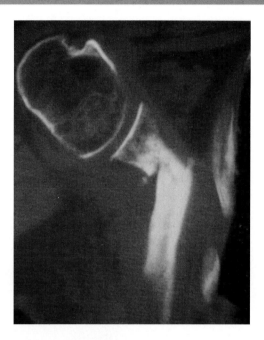
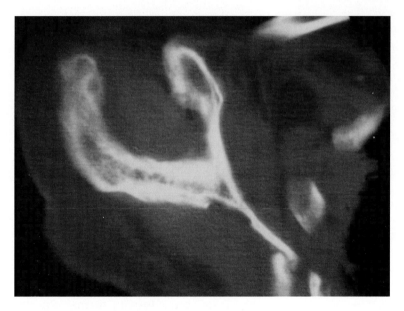

1. Describe the findings.

2. Why is this condition not Paget's disease?

3. What is the latent period between radiation therapy and development of radiation osteitis, provided a sufficient dose has been administered?

4. Why is the incidence of nonunion so high in patients with radiation-induced pathologic fractures of the shoulder?

Radiation Osteitis

1. Localized osteopenia, coarse trabeculation in the scapula and ribs, localized cortical thickening in the scapula and ribs, focal cortical lysis, and pathologic fractures of the scapula and ribs.

2. Involvement of the ribs is very uncommon for Paget's disease. In the scapula, Paget's disease tends to affect the acromion process and the coracoid process.

3. Minimum of 1 year.

4. Many fractures do not elicit symptoms, so patients are not immobilized.

Reference

Libshitz HI: Radiation changes in bone. Semin Roentgenol 29:15-37, 1994.

Comments

Radiation osteitis defines a spectrum of pathologic findings that occur in the bone after exposure to radiation. The changes are proportional to the dose administered. These findings include transient growth arrest, periostitis, bone sclerosis with increased fragility, ischemic necrosis, and infectious osteonecrosis. It is caused by a combination of damage to the vessels that supply the bone and direct injury to the osteoblasts. A narrow zone of transition with the adjacent normal bone demarcates the radiation field. These changes are usually evident within 24 months, but a delayed reaction that occurs years after radiation therapy is not considered unusual.

The shoulder girdle is a frequent site of radiation in patients who have been treated for breast cancer. The typical appearance of an irradiated shoulder is osteopenia of the bones associated with coarsening of the trabeculae and cortical lysis involving the scapula, clavicle, and ribs. Cortical thickening and osteosclerosis mimicking Paget's disease are less common manifestations. Pathologic fractures of the ribs and clavicle are common, and when these bones are fractured they frequently undergo resorption. Scapular fractures usually do not resorb but instead progress to nonunion. It is useful to note that when fractures are present, so are the radiographic features of osteitis. The differential diagnosis includes disuse osteoporosis, recurrent malignancy, and infection. The absence of periostitis or a soft-tissue component should be helpful in excluding the latter two diagnostic possibilities.

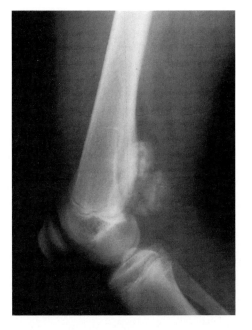
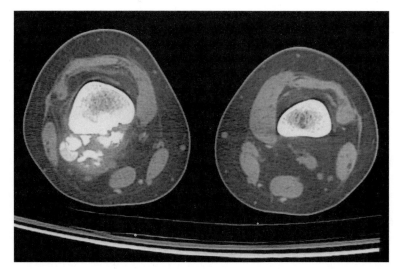

1. What is the differential diagnosis?
2. Is periostitis a typical feature of this neoplasm?
3. How do you think this lesion will be treated?
4. Why is magnetic resonance imaging (MRI) useful in staging malignant neoplasms?

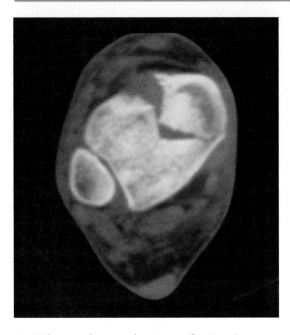
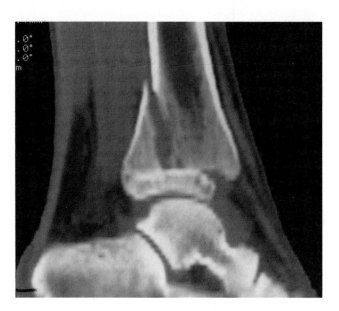

1. What is the mechanism of injury?
2. What determines whether the injury will result in a two-part or a three-part fracture?
3. How is this fracture different from a Tillaux fracture?
4. When assessing intra-articular fractures, how much incongruity is considered unacceptable?

C A S E 8 6

Parosteal Osteogenic Sarcoma

1. Myositis ossificans, parosteal osteosarcoma, juxtacortical chondroma and chondrosarcoma, and osteochondroma.

2. No.

3. Wide, regional, en bloc resection with limb salvage and chemotherapy.

4. Tumor extension can be characterized, particularly bone marrow invasion and extension into soft tissue.

References

Smith J, Ahuja SC, Huvos AG, Bullough PG: Parosteal (juxtacortical) osteogenic sarcoma. A roentgenological study of 30 patients. J Can Assoc Radiol 29:167–174, 1978.

Yu JS, Weis LD: MR imaging of parosteal osteosarcoma in two skeletally immature patients. Clin Imaging 21:63–68, 1997.

Comments

A parosteal osteogenic sarcoma (POS) is a slow-growing malignant tumor of bone arising from the periosseous tissues adjacent to the cortex. It accounts for 1.7% of all bone tumors and 4% of all osteosarcomas. The most common location is around the knee (70% of cases), with a predilection for the posterior surface of the distal femur. Generally, medical attention is sought after a long duration of symptoms, which include localized or painful swelling, development of a mass, joint dysfunction, or joint pain. This tumor can metastasize or invade the bone marrow, but POS has a relatively good prognosis if it is detected before significant extension into the medullary cavity. POS is frequently detected in the third and fourth decades of life, although 10% to 25% of lesions occur in patients who are younger than 19 years.

The characteristic radiographic appearance of POS is an osteoblastic, exophytic, broad-based mass arising from the surface of the bone. As it enlarges, the tumor has a tendency to encircle the bone, resulting in a thin radiolucent zone that separates the tumor from the underlying bone. The cortex usually does not become invaded until late in the course of the disease. When staging a POS, it may be preferable to use both computed tomography (CT) and MRI. MRI is recommended for assessment of the bone marrow and surrounding soft tissues, whereas CT is optimal for assessment of cortical integrity.

C A S E 8 7

Triplane Fracture

1. External rotation of the ankle, often with plantar flexion of the foot.

2. Age of patient (fusion of the growth plate).

3. A Tillaux fracture is a Salter type 3 fracture of the lateral tibial epiphysis.

4. Displacement exceeding 2 mm.

Reference

Ovadia DN, Beals RK: Fractures of the tibial plafond. J Bone Joint Surg Am 68:543–551, 1986.

Comments

The term *triplane fracture* refers to a fracture of the distal tibia that occurs in skeletally immature patients. The lateral half of the distal tibial epiphysis and physeal plate and the posterior tibial metaphysis are involved. "Triplane" indicates that fractures occur in all three geometric planes. The fracture planes include a sagittally oriented fracture through the epiphysis, a transverse fracture through the anterolateral aspect of the physeal plate, and a coronally oriented oblique fracture through the posterior aspect of the metaphysis. There are two types of triplane fractures, and the appearance of the fracture is dependent on fusion of the medial portion of the growth plate. When the physeal plate is unfused, these fractures result in three fragments. Older adolescents, owing to their partially fused growth plate, develop a two-fragment triplane fracture because the medial malleolus remains attached to the tibial shaft.

Computed tomography is advocated for delineating the extent of injuries in patients with triplane fractures. It accurately identifies the number of fracture fragments and the degree of displacement of the epiphysis, and the reformatted images allow determination of any distraction of the growth plate. Articular incongruity that exceeds 2 mm requires reduction. Radiographically, these fractures mimic Salter-Harris type 4 fractures because they represent a combination of Salter type 2 fracture of the posterior tibial metaphysis and Salter type 3 fracture of the medial aspect of the distal tibial epiphysis.

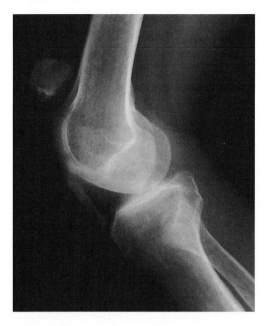

1. Describe two common mechanisms that can cause rupture of the extensor mechanism.
2. List the structures that must be disrupted if a patient loses the ability to completely extend the injured knee.
3. What predisposes a tendon to rupture?
4. When did the injury occur in this patient?

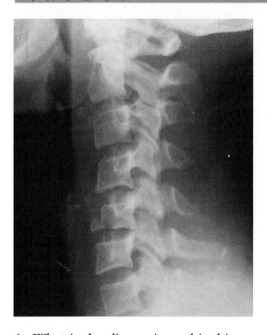

1. What is the diagnosis, and is this considered a stable or an unstable fracture?
2. Are neurologic deficits commonly seen in patients with this injury?
3. Why is this injury not a hyperextension injury?
4. What are indicators of instability?

Patellar Tendon Rupture

1. Rapid deceleration while running and quadriceps failure while ascending or descending stairs.

2. The quadriceps or patellar tendon and at least one of the patellar retinacula.

3. Repeated microtrauma (tendinosis) and systemic diseases (renal disease, crystal diseases such as gout and calcium pyrophosphate deposition, diabetes mellitus, rheumatoid arthritis, systemic lupus erythematosus, hyperparathyroidism).

4. A long time ago. Notice that the quadriceps muscles have atrophied and that heterotopic (dystrophic) ossification has developed in the patellar tendon.

Reference

Yu JS, Petersilge C, Sartoris DJ, et al: MR imaging of injuries of the extensor mechanism of the knee. Radiographics 14:541-551, 1994.

Comments

The extensor mechanism of the knee consists of tendons of the quadriceps femoris muscles, patella, patellar tendon, patellar retinacula, extensor hood, and insertion of the patellar tendon into the tibial tubercle. Normal tendons do not rupture under stress and are capable of withstanding up to 17.5 times normal body weight. Abnormally, tendons weakened by degeneration or repetitive microtrauma are susceptible to rupture. The common locations for these ruptures are at the enthesis of the tendon, and the inferior pole attachment of the patellar tendon is the most common location for failure of this tendon. In this patient, it is obvious that the injury occurred a long time ago. A sufficient length of time has passed to allow ossification of an intratendinous hematoma that developed within the patellar tendon, atrophy of the quadriceps muscles, and the patella's coming to rest in a high (alta) position from posttraumatic contraction of the quadriceps muscles. Acutely, this injury is treated with surgical repair before distraction occurs at the site of rupture.

Hyperflexion Teardrop (C5) Fracture

1. Hyperflexion teardrop fracture of C5 with a unilaterally locked facet at C5-C6. Unstable.

2. Yes, 75% to 90% of patients present with quadriplegia.

3. Fractures associated with hyperextension are usually small chip fractures from the anterior inferior aspect of the body.

4. Subluxation by more than 3 mm, angular deformity greater than 11 degrees, increased interspinous distance, widening of facet joints, narrowing of disk space, and compression of the vertebral body by more than 25%.

Reference

Kim KS, Chen HH, Russell EJ, Rogers LF: Flexion teardrop fracture of the cervical spine: Radiographic characteristics. AJR Am J Roentgenol 152:319-326, 1989.

Comments

Hyperflexion injuries of the cervical spine are caused by a direct blow against the top of the skull that results in forward arching of the head. The vector of the force is transmitted to the anterior aspect of the vertebral bodies. A hyperflexion teardrop fracture is considered the most unstable fracture of the cervical spine. It is associated with a high incidence of neurologic complications. On the lateral radiograph, one should look with suspicion at any kyphotic curvature of the cervical spine or abnormal widening of the interspinous distance (look at C4-C5). The most common location for this type of fracture is in the lower cervical spine. The triangular teardrop fragment usually involves the anterior and inferior aspects of the body, although it may also involve the anterior and superior aspects of the body in one sixth of cases. One of the critical steps in the evaluation of a patient with a hyperflexion injury is determining the integrity of the posterior ligaments, because disruption of these ligaments contributes significantly to instability. Subluxation may be obscured on a supine lateral view, so be careful. Upright views should eventually be performed.

Asymmetrical forces may result in angulation and rotation of the cervical spine. The radiographic manifestations of a unilaterally locked or perched facet joint may be subtle. Look for a change in the obliquity of the cervical spine occurring at the level of the injury. If both the lateral and the oblique radiographs appear simultaneously rotated and not rotated (we may think it is suboptimal), consider this diagnosis.

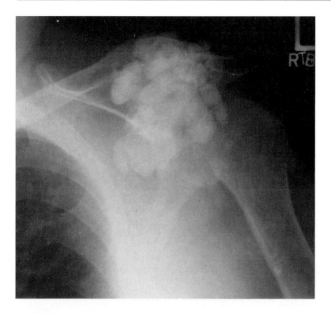
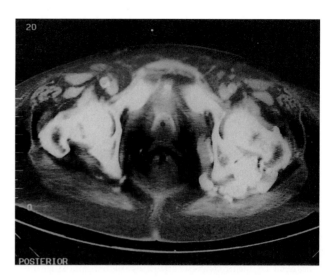

1. What is the differential diagnosis?
2. What information would help narrow the differential diagnosis?
3. List some causes of metastatic soft-tissue calcification (secondary tumoral calcinosis).
4. Are the hands commonly involved in idiopathic tumoral calcinosis?

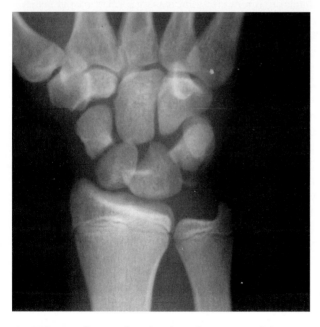
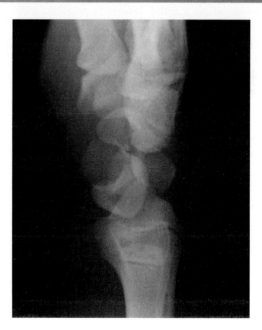

1. What radiographic landmarks are useful in assessing carpal stability?
2. What other osseous injuries may occur in this situation?
3. Why is this not volar intercalated segmental instability?
4. What would be an indication for magnetic resonance imaging? For computed tomography?

Idiopathic Tumoral Calcinosis

1. Idiopathic tumoral calcinosis, calcinosis universalis, metastatic calcification, and collagen vascular diseases such as dermatomyositis and scleroderma.

2. Age and ethnic background, underlying systemic disease, abnormal serum phosphate and calcium levels, symptoms (pain, swelling), number and size of affected joints, and distribution of soft-tissue calcification.

3. Hyperparathyroidism, hypoparathyroidism, renal osteodystrophy, hypervitaminosis D, milk-alkali syndrome, sarcoidosis, and processes associated with massive bony destruction such as metastasis.

4. No.

Reference

Steinbach LS, Johnston JO, Tepper EF, et al: Tumoral calcinosis: Radiologic-pathologic correlation. Skeletal Radiol 24:573–578, 1995.

Comments

Idiopathic tumoral calcinosis is a rare condition characterized by masslike deposits of calcium salts around joints. The cause of this disorder may be a defect in phosphate processing in the proximal renal tubules. The deposition of these calcific masses is painless and typically involves the shoulders, hips, and elbows. Patients affected are usually young, presenting between the ages of 6 and 25 years, and there is a strong affinity of the condition for black people. The calcium deposits are extracapsular in location and appear as radiodense masses surrounding a joint. The masses tend to enlarge from small, calcified nodules to large, solid, lobulated calcific lesions with smooth peripheral margins. The bony structures beneath these masses are usually normal. Occasionally, a fluid-fluid level may be evident in the region of dense calcifications. When the calcific masses are large, the range of motion of the adjacent joint may be limited and the overlying skin may break down, forming a sinus that drains a viscous, chalky material. Generally, no serum abnormality is evident, although, rarely, the alkaline phosphatase and phosphate levels may be elevated.

Trans-scaphoid Perilunate Dislocation

1. Intact proximal, middle, and distal arcuate Gilula's lines.

2. Fractures of the radial styloid, capitate, triquetrum, and ulnar styloid (greater arc injury pattern).

3. The lunocapitate articulation is dislocated.

4. Occult fracture, triangular fibrocartilage tears, instability. Intra-articular entrapment of osseous fragments.

References

Moneim M, Hofammann KE, Omer GE: Transscaphoid perilunate fracture-dislocation. Clin Orthop 190:227–235, 1984.

Yeager B, Dalinka M: Radiology of trauma to the wrist: Dislocations, fracture dislocations, and instability patterns. Skeletal Radiol 13:120–130, 1985.

Comments

The most common mechanism of injury is a fall on the palm of the hand resulting in hyperextension of the wrist. In this position, the dorsal cortex of the distal radial articular surface fixes the lunate in place and apposes the scaphoid waist. Certain patterns of injury, referred to as *lesser arc injuries,* present a spectrum of injuries that reflects an increasing level of carpal instability. A scapholunate dissociation with rotatory subluxation of the scaphoid is the most stable of these injuries. Failure of the radiocapitate ligament causes perilunate instability, which leads to a perilunate dislocation. Further disruption of the volar radiotriquetral ligament destabilizes the triquetrolunate joint. Complete disruption of the radiocarpal ligaments allows complete dislocation of the lunate.

Greater arc injuries represent a spectrum of fracture-dislocation patterns where the injury arc traverses through the scaphoid, capitate, hamate, and triquetrum. A trans-scaphoid perilunate dislocation (de Quervain's fracture-dislocation) is one such injury. In this injury, the lunate and the proximal pole of the scaphoid remain nearly aligned with the distal radius, whereas the carpus and the distal scaphoid fragment displace dorsally. Confirmation of adequate reduction of the scaphoid is critical on postreduction radiographs because any malalignment will impede fracture healing and may also promote instability.

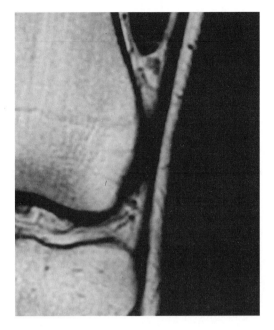
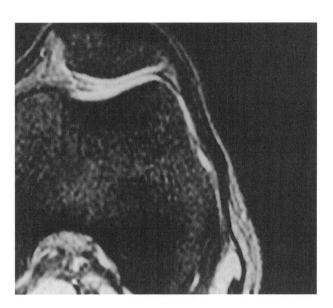

1. What is the most likely diagnosis in this runner?
2. What is the cause of this overuse syndrome?
3. How do these patients present clinically?
4. List some contributing factors that lead to the development of this syndrome.

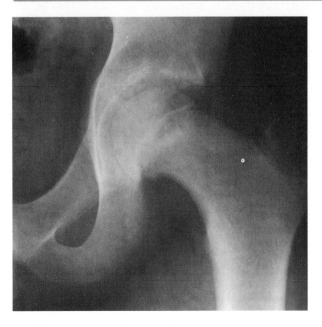
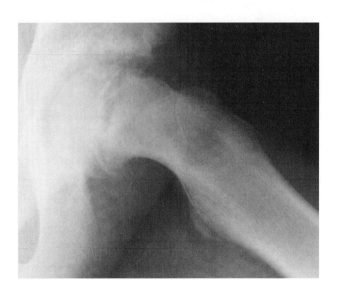

1. What is your diagnosis?
2. When do these patients usually present?
3. Although the cause is unknown, what are several predisposing conditions?
4. What is the aim of treatment? What is considered the treatment of choice?

Iliotibial Band Friction Syndrome

1. Iliotibial band (ITB) friction syndrome.

2. Irritation of the iliotibial tract (ITT) from constant rubbing against the femur during repeated flexion and extension of the knee.

3. Lateral joint pain over the epicondylar prominence of the lateral femoral condyle.

4. Large lateral epicondylar prominence, taut ITT, genu varum, or excessive internal rotation of the tibia.

Reference

Kavanaugh J, Yu JS: Too much of a good thing: Overuse injuries in the knee. Magn Reson Imaging Clin N Am 8:321-334, 2000.

Comments

The ITB friction syndrome is an overuse syndrome caused by irritation of the ITT when it repeatedly rubs over the epicondylar prominence of the distal femur during knee flexion and extension. A typical patient with ITB friction syndrome participates in an activity that requires constant knee flexion, such as long-distance running or cycling. Patients experience pain that localizes to a small area over the lateral femoral condyle just proximal to the lateral joint line. The differential diagnosis often includes a lateral meniscal tear, an injury to the lateral collateral ligament, and pathology of the popliteal tendon. On physical examination, common findings are tenderness and swelling over the lateral epicondylar prominence and crepitus, and the patient may exhibit a positive "compression" test result, pain that is induced by active motion of the knee while pressure is exerted by an examiner over the lateral femoral condyle.

The diagnosis of ITB syndrome is readily apparent on magnetic resonance imaging. These patients reveal a fluid collection or edema in the soft tissues deep to the ITT, either directly over or slightly posterior to the epicondylar prominence of the lateral femoral condyle. Patients may also present with signal abnormalities consistent with edema in the subcutaneous fat superficial to the ITT. In general, the ITT maintains normal signal intensity, although on rare occasion the posterior fibers of the ITT, the region of the ITT that is under greater tension, can appear edematous. Thickening of the ITT is a finding that is compatible with chronic disease.

Slipped Capital Femoral Epiphysis

1. Slipped capital femoral epiphysis (SCFE) of the left hip.

2. Between the ages of 10 and 17 years, with a peak incidence of 13 years in boys and 12 years in girls.

3. Trauma, obesity, hormonal abnormalities such as hypothyroidism, rapid growth spurts, renal osteodystrophy, and poor nutrition.

4. Restoring fusion of the growth plate. Pinning the epiphysis with minimal reduction.

Reference

Reynolds RA: Diagnosis and treatment of slipped capital femoral epiphysis. Curr Opin Pediatr 11:80-83, 1999.

Comments

SCFE is a childhood disorder of the hip characterized by posterior and inferior displacement of the proximal femoral epiphysis. It is usually a unilateral process, although 20% to 30% of cases are bilateral. Histologically, the abnormality occurs through the zone of hypertrophy in the growth plate. Clinically, patients present with poorly localized pain and a limp. The key to making the diagnosis is having both anteroposterior and frog-leg lateral radiographs available. This patient demonstrates classic findings. The cartilaginous growth plate is widened, and there is irregularity and rarefaction of the metaphysis. Close scrutiny of the frog-leg lateral projection often reveals that the initial direction of slippage is in the posterior direction, whereas the frontal radiograph may appear normal. As slippage progresses, the femoral epiphysis displaces medially, concomitantly widening the growth plate. SCFE may be classified according to the duration of symptoms or the degree of slippage. Patients are considered to have acute slips when symptoms have been present for less than 3 weeks. When symptoms last more than 3 weeks, this indicates a more chronic condition, associated with the development of characteristic radiographic abnormalities. The most severe consequence of SCFE is chondrolysis caused by pannus-like granulation tissue that erodes the articular cartilage. This complication predisposes the patient to secondary osteoarthritis.

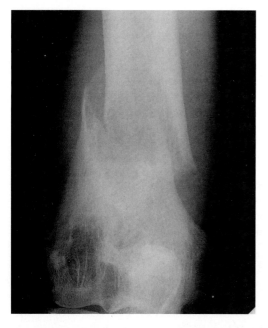 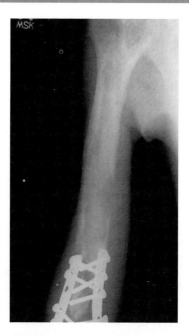

1. These images were obtained 8 months apart. What is your diagnosis?

2. When there is sarcomatous transformation, what are the common cell types? What are the prognoses?

3. Is this patient's radiographic presentation common?

4. When a giant cell tumor occurs in pagetic bone, where is it most likely to occur? What is the prognosis? Can it be multiple?

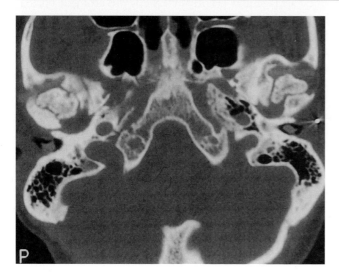 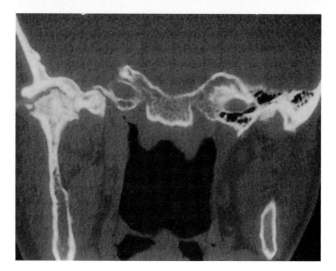

1. What is the disease process?

2. How is this condition treated?

3. Why is this not crystal deposition arthropathy?

4. What defines internal derangement of the temporomandibular joint?

Sarcomatous Transformation in Pagetic Bone

1. Sarcomatous transformation.

2. Osteosarcoma (50% to 60%), fibrosarcoma (20% to 25%), chondrosarcoma (10%). All poor.

3. Yes, osteolysis is the most common manifestation of sarcomatous degeneration and often causes a pathologic fracture.

4. In the skull or facial bones. Good. Yes.

Reference

Moore TE, King AR, Kathol MH, et al: Sarcoma in Paget disease of bone: Clinical, radiologic, and pathologic features in 22 cases. AJR Am J Roentgenol 156:1199–1203, 1991.

Comments

The diagnosis is not difficult once you realize that this patient has Paget's disease. Sarcomatous transformation is a well-described complication of Paget's disease. It is most common in elderly patients older than 60 years and occurs in about 1% of patients with Paget's disease. The most common locations for sarcomatous transformation are the femur, pelvis, and humerus. The most characteristic finding is osteolysis causing focal destruction of the bone. Other typical findings include a soft-tissue mass, disruption of the cortex, bony spiculation, and lack of a healing response in a persistent fracture. Lesions may be solitary or multifocal. Multicentric tumors have an extremely poor prognosis. It is important to remember that metastasis may also affect pagetic bone, especially that from the breast, lung, kidney, prostate, and colon. In these patients, you must look for other lesions in bone uninvolved with Paget's disease before you can dismiss malignant transformation from further consideration.

Silicone-Induced Arthritis

1. Silicone-induced arthropathy.

2. Removal of the silicone implant.

3. Silicone rubber is less radiodense than bone or calcium, and chondrocalcinosis is rare in the temporomandibular joint.

4. The location of the posterior band of the disk.

Reference

Goldman AB, Bansal M: Amyloidosis and silicone synovitis: Updated classification, updated pathophysiology, and synovial articular abnormalities. Radiol Clin North Am 34:375–394, 1996.

Comments

The use of silicone implants for repair of small joints was relatively common before the last decade, when they were used as spacers between the bones after resection surgery. However, some people developed a destructive arthropathy caused by the development of a foreign-body reaction, and this complication was an important factor in curtailing the use of silicone implants. The pathologic process begins when giant cells phagocytize the silicone particles that are released into the joint. This elicits an inflammatory cascade characterized by synovial hyperplasia and a giant cell infiltrate. The synovitis causes extensive destruction of the hyaline cartilage and eventually erodes the articular cortex and subchondral bone. Irreversible joint space loss, osseous fragmentation, and joint destruction are end-stage findings of silicone-induced arthritis, which is demonstrated in this patient. The key to the problem is how to determine the diagnosis early in the disease process. Notice the extruded fragments of silicone rubber anterior to and lateral to the joint. Initially, well-defined bone cysts filled with the silicone debris develop, and in most cases this finding precedes joint space loss. Transient periarticular demineralization should also alert you to the presence of a hyperemic response from the synovitis.

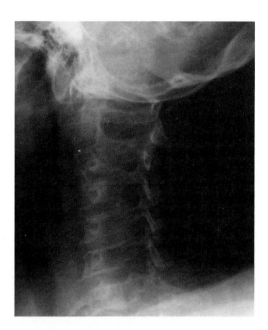 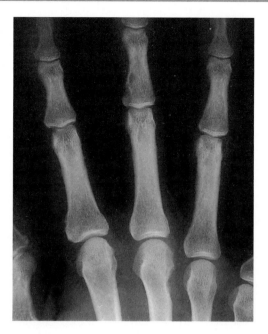

1. What do you think is the most likely diagnosis?

2. What did you observe in the spine radiograph? List the entities that you considered.

3. How does a schwannoma differ from a neurofibroma? Is it important for this patient to have this histologic distinction?

4. What observations did you make on the hand radiograph?

Neurofibromatosis

1. Neurofibromatosis.

2. Enlarged C2–C3 neural foramen. Neurofibroma, schwannoma, meningioma, and metastasis.

3. A schwannoma is a neural tumor of nerve sheath origin, and a neurofibroma is a tumor of nerve root or peripheral nerve origin. Yes, a neurofibroma likely indicates that the patient has neurofibromatosis 1, whereas a schwannoma would likely indicate that the patient has neurofibromatosis 2.

4. Pressure erosions of the head of the third metacarpal bone and the base of the middle phalanx from periosteal neurofibromas.

Reference

Shu HH, Mirowitz SA, Wippold FJ 2d: Neurofibromatosis: MR imaging findings involving the head and spine. AJR Am J Roentgenol 160:159–164, 1993.

Comments

Neurofibromatosis is a hereditary dysplasia that affects all three germ layers. It is transmitted as an autosomal dominant trait, although a family history is present in only 50% of cases. Other cases represent spontaneous mutations. Skin lesions are the most constant feature of neurofibromatosis, with café-au-lait spots occurring in 90% of patients. An elevated epidermal mass, called molluscum fibrosum, is another common skin lesion. A flat or domelike nodule in the iris of the eye (Lisch nodule) is common in patients older than 5 years.

The skeletal manifestations of neurofibromatosis are often the result of direct pressure from an adjacent tumor; however, dysplastic changes may involve the tibia, fibula, and clavicles, in the form of pseudoarthroses and bowing deformities. Acute angled scoliosis, particularly when it involves the upper thoracic spine, is characteristic of this disorder. In the ribs, dysplastic changes may result in a ribbon-like deformity, although intercostal neurofibromas may produce similar erosive changes. In this patient, a dumbbell-shaped neurofibroma exiting through the C2–C3 neural foramen caused marked widening of the foramen. This abnormality can be very pronounced in the cervical spine. The cystic lesions in the bones of the hand were caused by periosteal neurofibromas. Remember that not all bone lesions are neurofibromas. A well-marginated lytic lesion in the metaphysis of a bone may represent a nonossifying fibroma.

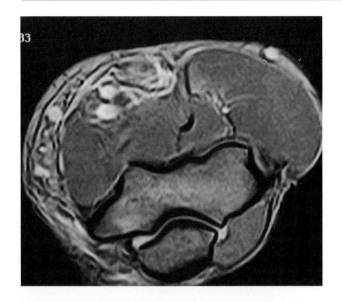
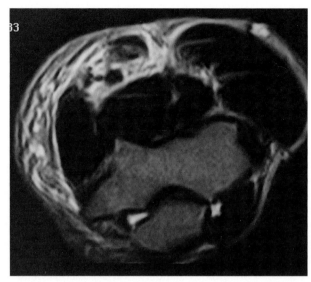
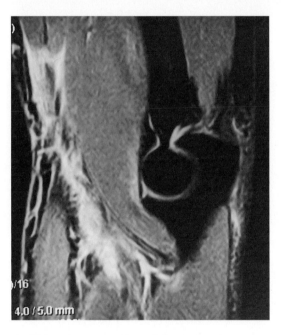

1. What happened to this patient?

2. How is this injury sustained?

3. In which direction does the biceps brachii muscle retract when it ruptures?

4. Where do most biceps tendon failures occur, at the insertion or at the musculotendinous junction?

Biceps Tendon Rupture

1. Rupture of the biceps tendon from the bicipital tuberosity of the proximal radius.

2. Forced hyperextension of a flexed elbow or forced flexion against resistance.

3. Proximally.

4. At the radial insertion.

Reference

Jorgensen U, Hinge K, Rye B: Rupture of the distal biceps brachii tendon. J Trauma 26:1061–1062, 1986.

Comments

The biceps brachii muscle originates from two locations on the scapula, the supraglenoid tubercle and the tip of the coracoid process, and inserts on the bicipital tuberosity of the proximal radius. Its primary action is flexion of the elbow joint, but it also contributes to supination of the forearm. Magnetic resonance imaging is the preferred method for evaluating rupture of the biceps tendon. When it occurs, patients complain of a tearing sensation and pain in the antecubital space, most frequently when lifting a heavy object. On examination, there is ecchymosis of the anterior arm about the elbow, tenderness in the antecubital fossa, and proximal retraction with flexion of the elbow. Weakening of elbow flexion and supination are notable findings.

On magnetic resonance imaging, the abnormality may be observed in the coronal, sagittal, and transaxial planes. On sagittal images, there is often a gap between the avulsed tendon and bicipital tuberosity. On T2W images, edema in and around the tendon may be noted, and the gap may be filled with fluid. On transaxial images, absence of the distal tendon just proximal to the bicipital tuberosity and interstitial edema in the soft tissues confirm the diagnosis. More proximally, there may be intense edema around a thickened tendon between the brachioradialis and brachialis muscles, anterior to the supinator muscle. Treatment is primary reattachment of the biceps tendon to the tuberosity within the first few days after the injury.

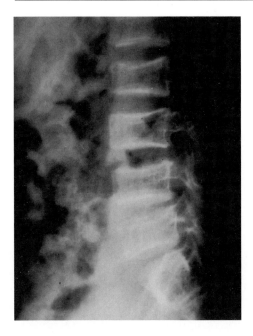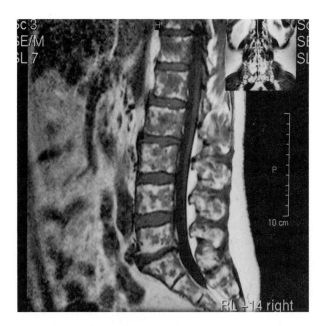

1. These two young adults have the same disease. What is the major radiographic observation? And on magnetic resonance imaging?

2. Describe a chloroma. What is its effect on the bone?

3. What arthropathy is a common complication of chronic leukemia?

4. Define reconversion of marrow.

Leukemia

1. Mild compression fractures in markedly osteopenic vertebral bodies. Diffuse marrow infiltration.

2. Soft-tissue masses composed of leukemic cells. These masses can produce osseous erosion.

3. Gout.

4. Transformation of inactive yellow marrow to active red marrow when there is an increased requirement for peripheral red blood cells and when the hematopoietic system is stressed or replaced.

Reference

Pear BL: Skeletal manifestations of the lymphomas and leukemias. Semin Roentgenol 9:229–240, 1974.

Comments

The key observation on the magnetic resonance image is diffuse marrow infiltration manifested by intermediate signal intensity throughout the spine on the T1W image. In the normal adult, the marrow distribution in the spine is relatively homogeneous, reflecting the different components of the bone marrow. The radiograph (both patients had acute myelocytic leukemia) identified an important observation, osteopenia in severely infiltrated marrow, and the magnetic resonance image shows diffuse skeletal involvement.

Leukemia is an infiltrative marrow disease characterized by neoplastic proliferation of one of the blood-forming cells. It can be classified as either acute or chronic depending on the duration of the disease. Skeletal involvement is present in nearly every case, although detectable osseous changes are conspicuous in only 75% of patients. Acute leukemia in adults may be associated with bone pain and tenderness, which is most common in the spine and the thoracic cage. Radiographically, bone changes in the adult are less frequent and less pronounced than in children. Generalized loss of bone density is a primary feature, although occasionally one may detect discrete osteolytic lesions (particularly in the skull, pelvis, and proximal long bones) and radiolucent metaphyseal bands (about 7% of cases). The presence of diffuse osteolytic lesions may mimic multiple myeloma. Periostitis, destructive lesions, and osteosclerosis are considered rare in an adult with acute leukemia but are more likely to occur in patients with chronic leukemia.

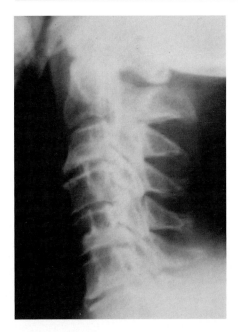
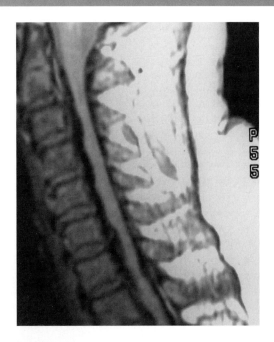

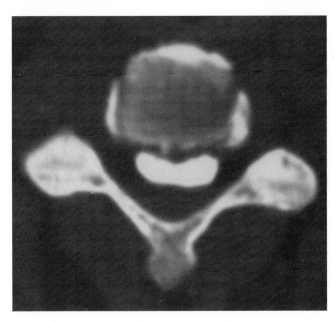

1. How would this patient present?

2. When do you expect cord signs (disturbances in motor and sensory function in the lower extremity) to be exhibited?

3. How often can you detect anterior vertebral osteophytes in patients with this condition?

4. Can this disorder occur elsewhere? How may the patients present?

Ossification of the Posterior Longitudinal Ligament

1. With neurologic symptoms or pain in the neck, shoulder, and upper extremity.

2. When the thickness of the ligament exceeds 60% of the sagittal diameter of the cervical spinal canal.

3. In about 30% to 50% of cases.

4. Yes, it may occasionally affect the thoracic (T4–T7) and lumbar (L1–L2) spine. With urinary and rectal incontinence.

References

Heller JG, Johnston RB 3d, Goodrich A: Ossification of the posterior longitudinal ligament: A report of nine cases in non-oriental patients. Skeletal Radiol 23:601–606, 1994.

Ono K, Yonenobu K, Miyamoto S, Okada K: Pathology of ossification of the posterior longitudinal ligament and ligamentum flavum. Clin Orthop 359:18–26, 1999.

Comments

Ossification of the posterior longitudinal ligament (OPLL) is a distinct clinical entity characterized by the development of ossifications, either in the form of a dense strip of bone or of small plaques, in the posterior longitudinal ligament. The majority of patients are middle-aged, and there is a 2:1 male-to-female ratio. Symptoms associated with this disorder have been related to cord impingement resulting in motor and sensory disturbances in either the lower or the upper extremity. Patients may also present with pain in the neck, shoulder, or arm, and possibly with neck stiffness. This case is an "aunt Minnie" and shows typical features of this condition. The ossification of the posterior longitudinal ligament is depicted as a dense strip of bone bridging the posterior aspect of the vertebral bodies from the C2 level to the C6 level (it occurs most frequently from C3 to C5). At the C4–C5 level, it narrows the diameter of the spinal canal by more than 50%. The cause of OPLL is unknown, although several factors have been suggested. The disorder frequently coexists in patients with diffuse idiopathic skeletal hyperostosis; however, there are distinct pathologic differences between the two entities.

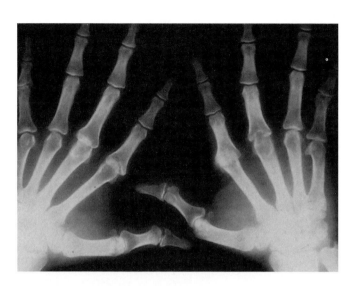
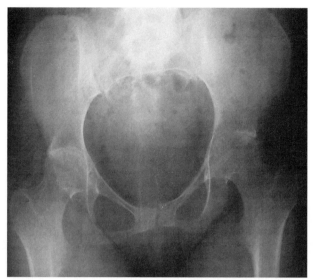

1. What is classic Still's disease?
2. What caused the "cupping" deformities of the proximal phalanges of the index and middle fingers?
3. Define Grisel's syndrome.
4. Can apophyseal joint ankylosis occur in both Still's disease and juvenile-onset ankylosing spondylitis?

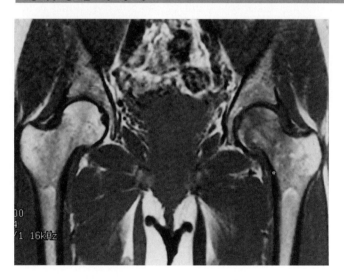
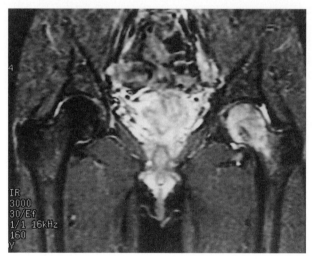

1. What is the differential diagnosis?
2. What will a joint aspiration reveal?
3. Can this condition recur and affect other joints? If so, what other joints may be affected, and what is this condition called?
4. What does bone scintigraphy show initially (when the patient is acutely symptomatic)?

Juvenile Chronic Arthritis

1. Pauciarticular or polyarticular disease, negative serologic tests for rheumatoid factor, and systemic manifestations such as fever, rash, weight loss, lymphadenopathy, and hepatosplenomegaly. In severe cases, pericarditis and myocarditis may be evident, as well as pleuritis and interstitial pulmonary disease.

2. Epiphyseal compression fractures from osteoporosis.

3. Nontraumatic atlantoaxial subluxation secondary to a retropharyngeal infection.

4. Yes.

References

Petersson H, Rydholm U: Radiologic classification of joint destruction in juvenile chronic arthritis. Acta Radiol 26:719-722, 1985.

Reiter MF, Boden SD: Inflammatory disorders of the cervical spine. Spine 23:2755-2766, 1998.

Comments

Children who present with arthritis have a condition that belongs to a group of disorders referred to as juvenile chronic arthritides. This group of diseases includes juvenile onset adult-type rheumatoid arthritis and Still's disease, which may be difficult to distinguish initially from juvenile-onset ankylosing spondylitis, psoriatic arthritis, and enteropathic arthritis. Still's disease constitutes the largest subgroup of juvenile chronic arthritis, and these patients present with pauciarticular or polyarticulardisease, absent serologic tests for rheumatoid factor, and systemic manifestations. The classic systemic subtype occurs in patients younger than 5 years and is associated with severe extra-articular manifestations. In the polyarticular subtype (the diagnosis in this patient), patients present later in life. The initial stages of polyarthritis are characterized by soft-tissue swelling, periarticular osteoporosis, periostitis, and advanced skeletal maturation. Epiphyseal overgrowth, associated with a gracile diaphysis, is a prominent finding and tends to be very noticeable in large joints. Joint space loss and erosive changes can lead to severe deformity and ankylosis of joints. Erosions are often preceded by epiphyseal compression fractures. In the cervical spine, which may be involved early, apophyseal joint erosions and narrowing and bony ankylosis are prominent features. Hypoplasia of the vertebral bodies and intervertebral disks is a distinctive finding. The most common subtype of Still's disease is the monoarticular or pauciarticular subtype, which comprises 30% to 70% of all patients with juvenile chronic arthritis. The large joints such as the knees, ankles, elbows, and wrists are typically affected. The hips and the small joints of the hands may be spared. Systemic manifestations are uncommon, but iridocyclitis may lead to blindness.

Transient Osteoporosis of the Hip

1. Acute osteonecrosis, transient osteoporosis of the hip, transient bone marrow edema syndrome.

2. Sterile effusion.

3. Yes. Knee, foot, and ankle—regional migratory osteoporosis.

4. Uptake of radionuclide tracer (occurs before development of osteopenia).

References

Bloem JL: Transient osteoporosis of the hip: MR imaging. Radiology 167:753-755, 1988.

Hays CW, Conway WF, Daniel WW: MR imaging of bone marrow edema pattern: Transient osteoporosis, transient bone marrow edema syndrome, or osteonecrosis. Radiographics 13:1001-1011, 1993.

Comments

Transient osteoporosis of the hip is a self-limiting condition characterized by pain in the hip that often radiates to the knee. It has a strong male predilection with a sex ratio of 3:1. It usually affects middle-aged men. In females, it often affects women who are in their third trimester of pregnancy. There is also a strong preponderance for involvement of the left hip. Initial radiographs may appear normal. However, as the disease progresses, osteopenia of the femoral head becomes evident. Diminished density of the femoral head demonstrates a characteristic loss of the outline of the articular cortical margin. The bone density in the acetabulum and femoral neck may also decrease, but this is usually less pronounced than in the femoral head. On magnetic resonance imaging (MRI), nonspecific bone marrow edema, manifested as regions of low signal intensity on T1W images and high signal intensity on T2W and inversion recovery images and involving the femoral head (sometimes extending to the femoral neck and intratrochanteric region) is seen without a demarcating region of osteonecrosis. An effusion is characteristically present.

The condition tends to regress without specific therapy over 2 to 4 months but may last as long as 9 months to 1 year. There is gradual reconstitution of the bone density, and, on follow-up MRI examinations, there is usually resolution of the bone marrow edema. The diagnostic considerations on MRI include early avascular necrosis, bone contusion, reflex sympathetic dystrophy, inflammatory arthritis, and osteomyelitis.

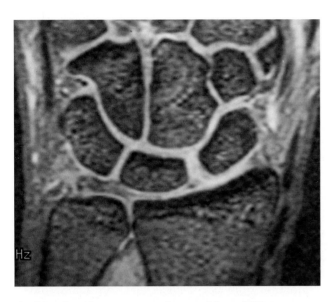
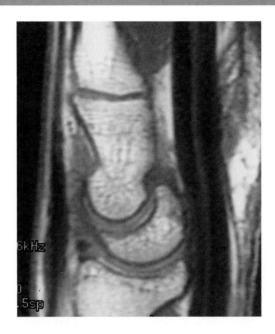

1. List the three types of carpal instability.

2. What are the two types of intercalary segmental instability patterns? Which is more common?

3. What are common causes of dorsal intercalated segmental instability (DISI)? Of volar intercalated segmental instability (VISI)?

4. List some causes other than trauma that result in carpal instability.

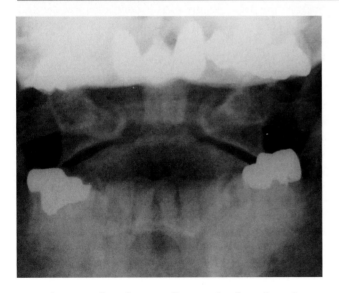
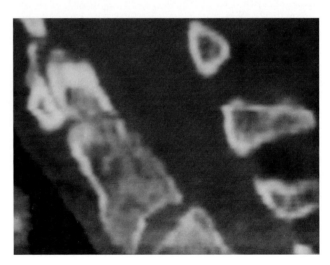

1. Where is the abnormality, and what does it mean with regard to treatment?

2. What does a small avulsion of the anteroinferior rim of the C2 body indicate?

3. How would you perform a computed tomography (CT) examination through the odontoid process?

4. What is a type 3 odontoid fracture, and is it stable or unstable?

Dorsal Intercalated Segmental Instability

1. Central column, medial column, and proximal.

2. Dorsal (DISI) and volar (VISI). DISI.

3. Scaphoid fractures, with disruption of the scapholunate ligament, and fracture of the distal radius. Disruption of the lunotriquetral ligament or midcarpal ligaments.

4. Ligamentous laxity, rheumatoid arthritis, and crystal deposition arthropathy (especially calcium pyrophosphate deposition).

Reference

Yeager B, Dalinka M: Radiology of trauma to the wrist: Dislocations, fracture dislocations, and instability patterns. Skeletal Radiol 13:120-130, 1985.

Comments

Carpal instability is an important sequela of ligamentous injury, and three important patterns should be recognized. The first pattern relates to abnormalities of the central column of the wrist, composed principally of the lunate and the capitate. In a normal situation, a continuous line can be drawn through the long axis of the radius, lunate, capitate, and third metacarpal bone. A normal lunocapitate (LC) angle is less than 20 degrees. An intersecting line drawn through the long axis of the scaphoid creates an angle (scapholunate [SL] angle) of 30 to 60 degrees. Intercalary segmental instability denotes disruption of the SL angle, the LC angle, or both. In DISI, shown here, the lunate tilts dorsally and the scaphoid is flexed so that the SL angle exceeds 70 degrees. In VISI, the lunate tilts volarly so that the SL angle is less than 47 degrees. In both situations, the LC angle exceeds 20 degrees, but in opposite directions.

The second pattern of instability involves the medial aspect of the carpus. There are two main types, triquetrohamate dissociation and triquetrolunate dissociation, indicating the pathologic motion between the carpal bones for which the dissociation is named. The last pattern is proximal carpal instability caused by disruption of the radiocarpal ligaments or the distal radioulnar joint. A fracture of the distal radius is an important factor that leads to the development of this type of instability.

Odontoid Fractures

1. Type 2 fractures are unstable and frequently lead to nonunion; therefore, they generally require a C1-C2 fusion.

2. Avulsion of the attachment of the anterior longitudinal ligament. May indicate a type 3 fracture.

3. Thin sections (1-mm sections with 0.5 mm of overlap) for optimal reformation of images. Remember that thicker slices may cause volume averaging of type 2 fractures.

4. Type 3 fractures occur through the cancellous portion of the bone and are considered stable because they heal well with conservative management using a halo device.

Reference

Anderson LD, D'Alonzo RT: Fractures of the odontoid process of the axis. J Bone Joint Surg Am 56:1663-1674, 1978.

Comments

Fractures of the odontoid process are usually the result of head trauma transmitted to the C1-C2 area. If the dens is displaced, its direction is dictated by the force that is transmitted. The most common classification is the Anderson and D'Alonzo classification, which describes three odontoid fracture types. In type 1, the fracture involves the tip of the odontoid process and most likely represents an avulsion by the alar ligaments. In type 2, the most common type, a fracture occurs at the base of the odontoid process or below the level of the superior articular facet of C2. In type 3, there is a fracture involving the body of C2. Generally, an odontoid fracture is not a difficult diagnosis to make if the lateral view is positioned well and an odontoid projection is adequate. However, CT is recommended for delineating the extent of injury and for assessing the insertion of the anterior longitudinal ligament. Thin-section CT with reformatted images is advocated because it also enables evaluation of the attachments of the alar and transverse ligaments, which can be indicators of an unstable situation if they are avulsed. More recently, magnetic resonance imaging has become more widely used for evaluating these fractures for the same reasons that popularized the use of CT.

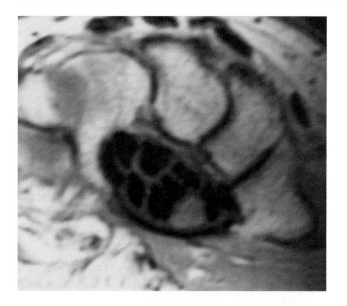

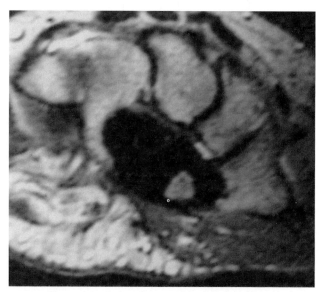

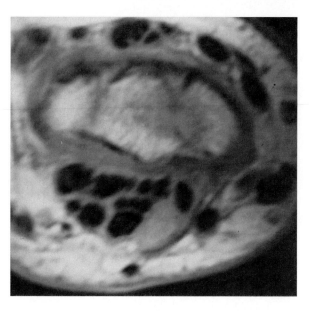

1. List the clinical manifestations of this condition.

2. What is a positive Tinel's sign? What is Phalen's test?

3. What other magnetic resonance imaging (MRI) findings are diagnostic of this disorder?

4. Does this patient have a pseudoneuroma? What is it?

Carpal Tunnel Syndrome

1. Nocturnal hand discomfort; paresthesia in the thumb and the second, third, and radial side of the fourth fingers; and weakness and atrophy of the thenar musculature.

2. Tingling in the digits supplied by the median nerve. Flex both wrists for 60 seconds—numbness in the median nerve distribution should occur within 60 seconds in the presence of carpal tunnel syndrome (CTS).

3. Compression, diffuse flattening, or an abrupt change in the morphology of the median nerve, edema of the nerve, or enhancement with gadolinium administration.

4. Yes, enlargement of the median nerve proximal to the carpal tunnel. Associated with constriction of the median nerve distal to the point of swelling.

Reference

Yu JS: Magnetic resonance imaging of the wrist. Orthopedics 17:1041-1048, 1994.

Comments

CTS is a common neuropathy of the upper extremity caused by compression of the median nerve in the carpal tunnel. It typically involves middle-aged women and presents as a bilateral condition in nearly half of those affected. Common causes of CTS include tenosynovitis, masses (ganglion or neuroma), synovial proliferation, and diminished girth of the carpal canal from posttraumatic osseous changes and fibrosis. Chronic hypoxia has also been suggested as a potential precipitating event. Most cases of CTS, however, are idiopathic and are likely the result of a normal aging process. MRI is useful for confirming the diagnosis of CTS in patients exhibiting symptoms. Characteristic findings are depicted on true transaxial images of the wrist and proximal hand. MRI findings diagnostic of CTS include compression and flattening of the median nerve, increased signal intensity in the median nerve on T2W images, bowing of the flexor retinaculum, loss of the normal fat between the carpal bones and the tendons, and an abrupt change of the diameter of the median nerve.

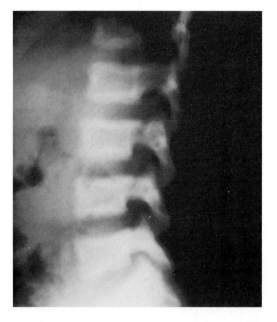
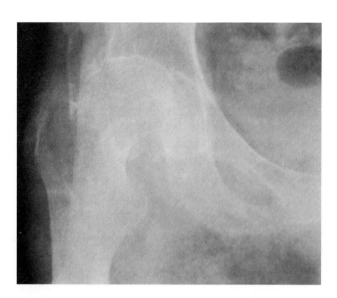

1. The first radiograph was obtained when the patient was an adolescent, whereas the second shows his hip about 15 years later. What may have been the etiology of his bone disorder?

2. What is the normal interval between osteoid synthesis and mineralization? What about in this patient?

3. What biochemical abnormality is associated with rickets?

4. Describe Fanconi's syndrome.

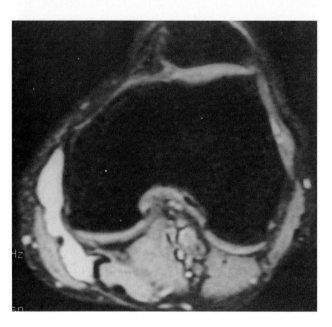
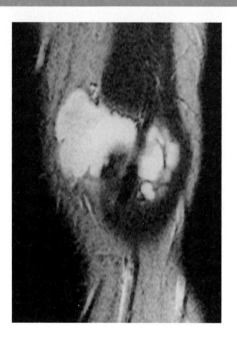

1. What is the pes anserinus?

2. What structure separates the pes anserinus from the tibial collateral ligament?

3. What entities did you consider in this patient? Where is a typical Baker's cyst found?

4. What does a fluid-fluid level in a popliteal cyst indicate?

Osteomalacia

1. Vitamin D deficiency, hypophosphatemia with adequate vitamin D, and defective nucleation without calcium, phosphorus, or vitamin D abnormalities.

2. Five to 10 days. More than 3 months.

3. Hypophosphatemia.

4. Defect in renal tubular resorption leads to excessive excretion of amino acids, phosphate, glucose, calcium, potassium, protein, and water.

References

Renton P: Radiology of rickets, osteomalacia and hyperparathyroidism. Hosp Med 59:399-403, 1998.

Reynolds WA, Karo JJ: Radiologic diagnosis of metabolic bone disease. Orthop Clin North Am 3:521-543, 1972.

Comments

Osteomalacia is a pathologic condition caused by the accumulation of uncalcified osteoid. Proper metabolism of vitamin D is required for healthy bones and muscles. Vitamin D metabolites affect the homeostasis of calcium and phosphorus. Patients with osteomalacia complain of muscular weakness, nonspecific pain, and weak bones that become deformed with time. There are numerous causes of osteomalacia, and you should be familiar with some of these. Causes include dietary deficiency of calcium or vitamin D, deficient absorption of calcium or phosphorus (conditions that cause malabsorption and obstructive jaundice), enzyme deficiencies, renal diseases (acquired and congenital), tumors, and liver disease.

The characteristic finding in osteomalacia is loss of bone density. Typical radiographic features include areas of mottled radiolucency and diminished trabeculation, coarsening of the remaining trabeculae, ill-defined cortices (especially endosteum), and changes in the morphology of the bone owing to softening and pseudofractures. In this patient, the bones appear "chalky." This is in contradistinction to osteoporosis, an entity caused by decreased osteoid production but normal mineralization. An osteoporotic spine demonstrates sharp cortical margins and prominent vertical trabeculation (owing to loss of horizontal trabeculae). Anterior wedging and central end-plate depression are characteristic bone deformities in osteoporotic patients, caused by compression fractures. This patient has developed a pseudofracture (Looser's line) in the medial aspect of the base of the femoral neck.

Pes Anserine Bursitis

1. A tripod of tendons (sartorius, gracilis, and semitendinosus) that insert on the posteromedial aspect of the proximal tibia.

2. Pes anserine bursa.

3. Meniscal cyst, ganglion, synovial cyst, and semimembranosus bursitis. Between the semimembranosus and medial gastrocnemius tendons.

4. Most likely a recent hemorrhage.

Reference

Forbes R, Helms CA, Janzen DL: Acute pes anserine bursitis: MR imaging. Radiology 194:525-527, 1995.

Comments

Numerous bursae are located about the knee. Any one of them may be subjected to repeated trauma, eliciting an inflammatory reaction when it has an intimate relationship with a tendon. The anserine bursa, which lies deep to the pes anserinus tendons, is a structure that may be traumatized from repeated flexion, extension, and rotation of the knee. Once inflammation has developed, the process may become a chronic condition, with symptoms persisting for months or even years. Clinically, patients complain of a burning sensation in the medial aspect of the knee that radiates down the calf. On physical examination, tenderness and swelling along the proximal aspect of the tibia are notable findings. Often, the differential diagnosis is either a tear of the medial meniscus or a strain of the medial collateral ligament, because climbing and descending stairs exacerbate the patient's symptoms.

The diagnosis is readily apparent on magnetic resonance imaging. The main finding is distention of the anserine bursa with fluid. The characteristic appearance is a collection of fluid deep to and often surrounding the semitendinosus tendon and located posterolaterally to the sartorius and gracilis tendons. Internal septations are common. When the bursitis is chronic, the fluid in the bursa is often of heterogeneous signal intensity, and the synovial lining may appear thickened. Erosive changes in the tibia also indicate a more chronic process.

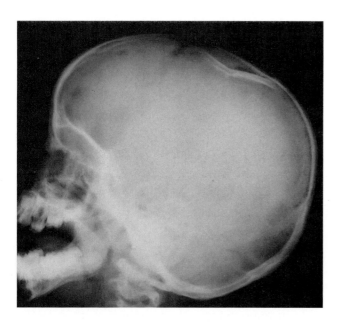
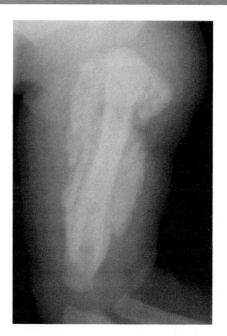
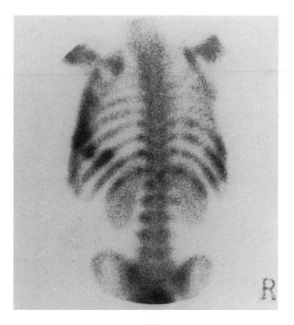

1. What is the diagnosis?
2. Why do subperiosteal hemorrhages occur in infants?
3. List some bony findings that would lead you to suspect child abuse.
4. Where do other manifestations of child abuse occur?

Battered Child Syndrome

1. Battered child syndrome (child abuse).

2. The periosteum and perichondrium are tightly attached at the terminal end of the metaphysis but loosely attached to the diaphysis.

3. Multiple and unusual fractures in different stages of healing, metaphyseal fragmentation, and subperiosteal hemorrhage with periostitis.

4. Skull—shaking injuries (subdural hematoma, intraventricular hemorrhage, subarachnoid hemorrhage, cerebral edema, and contusion). Abdomen—pancreatitis, liver contusions, perforations of gastrointestinal tract.

References

Mogbo KI, Slovis TL, Canady AI, et al: Appropriate imaging in children with skull fractures and suspicion of abuse. Radiology 208:521-524, 1998.

Neitzschman HR, McCarthy K: Radiology case of the month. Bruising of unknown etiology. Child abuse (the "battered child syndrome"). J La State Med Soc 150:11-12, 1998.

Comments

Abused children are at risk for sustaining life-threatening injuries, so it is incumbent on clinicians to recognize the radiographic and clinical signs that might indicate battered child syndrome. Metaphyseal fragmentation and cortical thickening without fractures or dislocations are common findings that should alert you to this diagnosis. The firm attachment of the periosteum to the metaphyses of tubular bones results in characteristic metaphyseal fragmentation that occurs immediately after trauma. The periosteum of a child is easily elevated by a subperiosteal hematoma when a tubular bone is traumatized. Reactive bone formation with sclerosis associated with periostitis is a compelling radiographic finding that should be apparent within 2 to 3 weeks after the injury. Skull fractures and widened cranial sutures are frequent injuries. Fractures in unusual locations, such as the sternum, scapula, lateral end of the clavicle, and vertebral bodies, should also arouse suspicion of abuse. Lower extremity fractures in infants who are not of walking age should be considered suspicious, especially if they are associated with overabundant callus formation. Multiple fractures, particularly involving the rib cage, require a careful search for other indications of child abuse. Bone scintigraphy is a useful adjunct to conventional radiographs. Single or multiple fractures, particularly of the ribs, humerus, femur, tibia, and small bones of the hands and feet, are strongly suggestive of abuse.

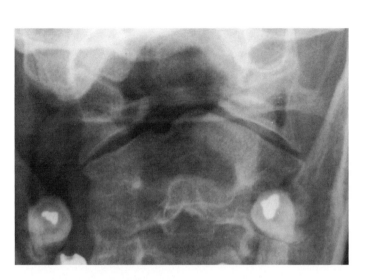
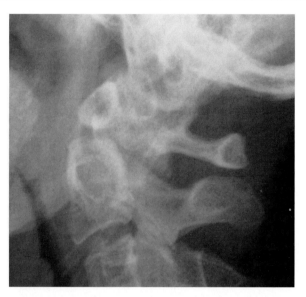

1. What is the diagnosis?
2. What determines atlantoaxial instability when this anomaly is observed?
3. Can this abnormality occur after trauma?
4. What other conditions can cause cortical thickening and hypertrophy of the anterior arch of C1?

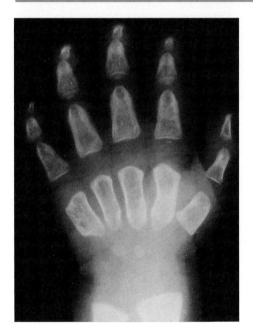
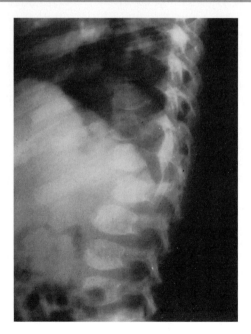

1. What is the differential diagnosis?
2. In general terms, what is the essential defect that results in these syndromes? What are the common excreted products?
3. What is different about Hunter's syndrome compared with other forms of mucopolysaccharidoses?
4. What is a "gargoyle cell" or a "clear cell"?

Os Odontoideum

1. An os odontoideum.

2. The juxtaposition of the transverse ligament of C1 to the ossicle.

3. Some cases actually represent nonunion of a type 2 odontoid fracture.

4. Chronic rheumatologic conditions such as osteoarthritis and rheumatoid arthritis.

Reference

Matsui H, Imada K, Tsuji H: Radiographic classification of os odontoideum and its clinical significance. Spine 22:1706–1709, 1997.

Comments

An os odontoideum is a small bone that exists above a hypoplastic odontoid process. It has a characteristic appearance: a small, round or oval, well-corticated ossicle located above the tip of the odontoid process or more cephalad near the basion of the skull. When evaluating this anomaly, one clue is to search for coexisting abnormalities of the atlas, including hypoplasia of the posterior neural arch and hypertrophy of the anterior arch. Most experts agree that an os odontoideum represents a congenital anomaly (overgrowth of the os terminale secondary to hypoplasia of the odontoid), although some cases do represent a posttraumatic condition. The importance of an os odontoideum is its association with atlantoaxial instability. Stability is dependent on the level of the cleft between it and the odontoid process and on the degree of development of the dens. If the transverse ligament is juxtaposed to the ossicle, then the odontoid process is unable to form a stable relationship with the atlas, a configuration that is conducive to atlantoaxial instability. In severe cases of instability, the caliber of the spinal canal can be significantly compromised. Assessment of stability is performed with flexion and extension lateral radiographs. It is important to quantify the degree of motion of the ossicle and the changes in the caliber of the spinal canal. When the stability is in doubt, computed tomography or magnetic resonance imaging is advocated for further evaluation of the integrity of the transverse ligament.

Hurler's Syndrome

1. Hurler's syndrome, Morquio's syndrome, or Sanfilippo's syndrome.

2. Lack of specific enzymes needed to break down the side chains of the mucopolysaccharide molecule. Heparan sulfate and dermatan sulfate.

3. Hunter's syndrome occurs only in males because it is transmitted as an X-linked recessive trait.

4. A cell distended with cytoplasmic polysaccharide deposits.

Reference

Schmidt H, Ullrich K, von Lengerke HJ, et al: Radiological findings in patients with mucopolysaccharidosis I H/S (Hurler-Scheie syndrome). Pediatr Radiol 17:409–414, 1987.

Comments

The mucopolysaccharidoses constitute a group of syndromes characterized by specific enzyme deficiencies that impair the breakdown of the side chains of the mucopolysaccharide molecule. These patients excrete a predominant mucopolysaccharide in their urine: heparan sulfate and dermatan sulfate (Hurler's, Hunter's); heparan sulfate (Sanfilippo's, Scheie's); keratan sulfate (Morquio's); and dermatan sulfate (Maroteaux-Lamy). Radiographically, the manifestations in the axial skeleton are sufficiently similar (with a couple of exceptions) to prevent specific diagnosis. The key to diagnosis lies in making observations in the appendicular skeleton and in the skull, where there is some variation between these disorders (albeit subtle variation between Hurler's syndrome and Morquio's syndrome).

In this patient, the hand radiograph is helpful in eliminating all but two of the mucopolysaccharidoses. In both Hurler's and Morquio's syndromes, there is thickening of the shaft of the metacarpal bones and tapering of the proximal ends, resulting in a characteristic "bullet" appearance. Angular deformities of the articular surfaces are common, especially in the wrist. The trabeculation appears coarse. The spine radiograph enables you to further narrow your diagnosis. In the spine, diffuse morphologic changes (universal vertebra plana, late; ovoid bodies, early) are typical findings. Early in life, an anterior beak may protrude from the vertebral body, and its location is helpful in differentiating among these processes: inferior (Hurler's, Hunter's), central (Morquio's), or both (Sanfilippo's).

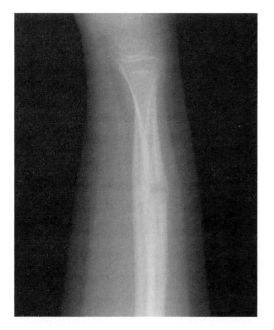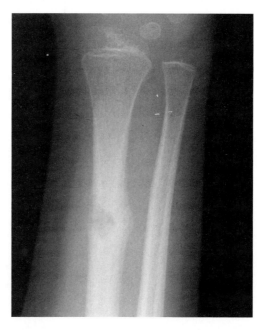

1. This patient presented with a pathologic fracture. What conditions would you consider?
2. How does the blood supply in the bones of children differ from that in the bones of adults?
3. What is a sequestrum?
4. How soon after the bone has been inoculated can you detect the formation of an involucrum?

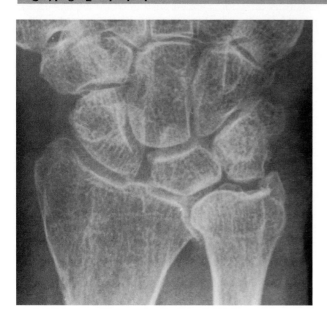

1. What soft-tissue structures are usually injured in this condition?
2. How is this condition treated?
3. What is ulnar variance?
4. Is variance static, or can it change?

Hematogenous Osteomyelitis

1. Osteomyelitis, metastasis, and, occasionally, Ewing's sarcoma.

2. In children, distinct epiphyseal and metaphyseal arteries are present on either side of the growth plate with little or no anastomoses between these vessels. The periosteum is more vascular, communicating freely with vessels in the shaft.

3. A fragment of dead bone in a region of infection.

4. Two weeks.

Reference

Gold R: Diagnosis of osteomyelitis. Pediatr Rev 12:292–297, 1991.

Comments

Hematogenous osteomyelitis is generally regarded as a disease of childhood. It affects the tubular bones of the lower extremity in 75% of cases. Clinically, the disease is associated with a sudden onset of fever and focal inflammation. In many instances, there is no systemic sign of infection, and suspicion is aroused only by the presence of soft-tissue swelling, diminished range of motion, or joint effusion. Bacteria (group B streptococci or *Staphylococcus aureus*) are the major cause of osteomyelitis in neonates and infants. The bacteria may be introduced by vascular catheterization, monitoring devices, and repeated venipuncture, eventually settling in the terminal capillaries of the metaphysis. Once in the bone, destruction and abscess formation ensue. From this location, bacteria are free to spread into the joint (hip), the medullary cavity (tubular bones), or the subperiosteal space, stripping the periosteum from the cortex. As the vascular supply becomes compromised, the bone dies.

Radiographically, the initial infectious process may be insidious. As the infection progresses, destructive changes in the bone develop, as does soft-tissue swelling. The main observation in this patient is a focal area of bone lysis in the diaphysis of the radius surrounded by laminated periostitis (involucrum) and endosteal new bone formation. A pathologic fracture is present, although this is not a common finding in patients of this age. If allowed to take its course, the infection would likely cause cortical necrosis and formation of a sequestrum.

Ulnar Impingement Syndrome

1. Articular hyaline cartilage, triangular fibrocartilage, and lunotriquetral ligament.

2. Ulnar length shortening and débridement of the triangular fibrocartilage perforation.

3. This term refers to the relative length of the radius and ulna. If the ulna is short, the variance is negative. If the ulna is long, the variance is positive. Neutral variance refers to equal lengths of the radius and ulna.

4. The position of the wrist can affect the ulnar variance. Supination causes relative ulnar shortening, whereas pronation causes relative lengthening.

Reference

Friedman SL, Palmer AK: The ulnar impaction syndrome. Hand Clin 7:295–310, 1991.

Comments

Ulnar impingement syndrome refers to a painful condition caused by compression of the distal ulna on the medial articular surface of the lunate. It is the result of a positive ulnar variance. The condition may be initiated by trauma. At its onset, there is little to no radiographic manifestation of the condition other than a long ulna. As the process becomes more chronic, flattening accompanied by areas of sclerosis may become evident in the articular surface of the lunate adjacent to the ulna. Pressure erosions may develop, resulting in cortical irregularity and cystic deformities. As the disease progresses, changes may also be noted in the triquetrum. In extreme cases of positive ulnar variance, the ulna subluxes dorsally, and supination is impeded. Magnetic resonance imaging is a useful technique for assessing the extent of injury to the triangular fibrocartilage. Central perforations of the triangular fibrocartilage are a common associated abnormality, as are degenerative changes of the meniscus. Diminished signal intensity in the bone marrow of the lunate corresponding to areas of subchondral sclerosis may be notable on both T1W and T2W coronal images, in addition to denudement of the overlying hyaline cartilage.

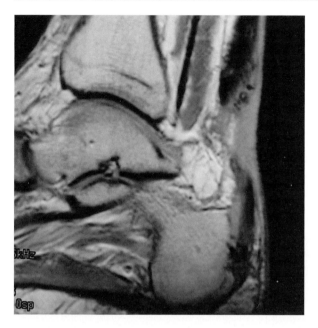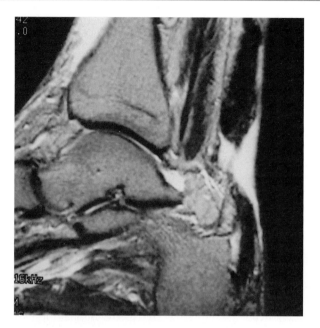

1. Where is the most common location for an Achilles' tendon rupture? Why?
2. Does the Achilles' tendon have a true tendon sheath? What other major tendon shares this similarity?
3. What is the Thompson test? How accurate is physical examination for a ruptured Achilles' tendon?
4. What determines if an injury is a surgical lesion?

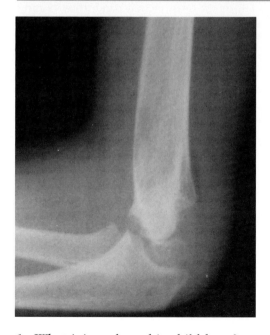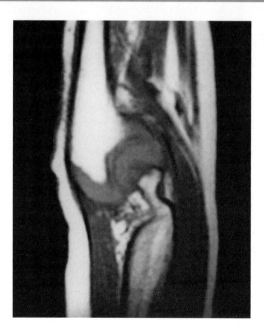

1. What injury does this child have?
2. Where should the capitellar ossification center be located with respect to the anterior humeral cortex?
3. Is this injury common? In what age group?
4. What is Bowman's angle, and what is it used to assess?

Achilles' Tendon Rupture

1. Approximately 2 to 6 cm above the insertion. Vascular watershed area.

2. No. Patellar tendon.

3. Squeezing the gastrocnemius muscle (with the patient in the prone position) does not produce normal plantar flexion. The accuracy is 75%.

4. Tears that rupture more than 50% of fibers, and patient's age and activity status.

Reference

Keene JS, Lash EG, Fisher DR, DeSmet AA: Magnetic resonance imaging of Achilles tendon ruptures. Am J Sports Med 17:333-337, 1989.

Comments

The Achilles' tendon is the largest tendon in the ankle, originating from the union of the gastrocnemius and soleus tendons and inserting on the posterior surface of the calcaneus. A rupture of this tendon is a severe injury and is caused by indirect trauma related to strenuous tensile forces. The majority of injuries are "pushing off" injuries with the foot in plantar flexion and the knee in extension, although a fall on the forefoot causing forced dorsiflexion of the foot can also injure the tendon. When a rupture occurs spontaneously, it tends to affect middle-aged people who have an underlying systemic disorder such as gout, chronic renal failure, diabetes mellitus, hyperparathyroidism, rheumatoid arthritis, and systemic lupus erythematosus. Patients present with acute-onset pain, ankle swelling, and an inability to rise on their toes.

On magnetic resonance imaging, a complete tear has a characteristic appearance on T2W images. High signal intensity (edema or hemorrhage) interposed between the frayed ends of the tendon is often associated with retraction and buckling of the proximal tendon fibers. On axial images, an "absent tendon" sign reflects images through the gap in the tendon. In partial tears, edema and hemorrhage may be confined to portions of the tendon, which may thicken in a fusiform fashion. It may be difficult to differentiate a chronically torn tendon from chronic tendinosis in the absence of ligamentous discontinuity.

Supracondylar Humerus Fracture

1. Supracondylar fracture of the humerus.

2. The anterior humeral line intersects the middle third of the capitellum.

3. Yes, it constitutes about 60% of elbow fractures in children. Between ages 4 and 10 years.

4. An angle formed by a line, which bisects the shaft of the humerus, subtended by a line formed along the metaphysis of the medial epicondyle. Used to assess the normal cubitus valgus angle of the elbow.

Reference

Minkowitz B, Busch MT: Supracondylar humerus fractures. Current trends and controversies. Orthop Clin North Am 25:581-594, 1994.

Comments

This patient shows classic findings of a supracondylar fracture of the distal humerus that was initially misdiagnosed as an elbow strain. You must recall that the metaphysis of the distal humerus and capitellum is anteverted about 140 degrees relative to the shaft of the humerus. Therefore, when a line is drawn along the anterior cortex of the humerus, it intersects the middle third of the capitellar ossification center (anterior humeral line). The majority of supracondylar fractures are caused by a fall on an outstretched hand, thus causing posterior displacement of the distal fracture fragment and disruption of the anterior humeral line. The fracture may also cause an abnormal cubitus varus or valgus angulation, which is identified when there is a discrepancy of 5 degrees or more between the injured elbow and the normal contralateral elbow. Magnetic resonance imaging is useful for evaluating patients with an incompletely ossified capitellum because it allows visualization of the cartilaginous ossification center.

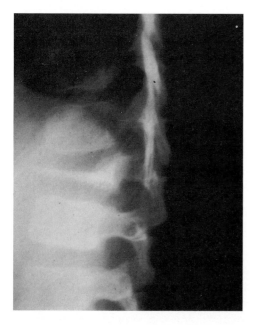

1. What is the most likely diagnosis, and what else did your differential diagnosis initially include?
2. Where is the most common location for an eosinophilic granuloma lesion?
3. Can you see this vertebral body morphology in achondroplasia?
4. What is the difference between vertebra plana and platyspondyly?

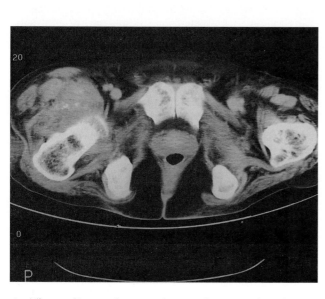 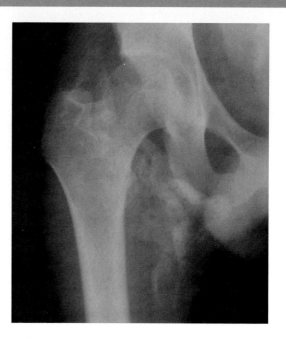

1. The radiograph was obtained 3 months after computed tomography (CT). What conditions would you consider if you had only the CT image?
2. What would you expect to see histologically?
3. Is periostitis common in this process?
4. Would the tissue enhance with administration of intravenous gadolinium?

Vertebra Plana

1. Eosinophilic granuloma. Metastasis, multiple myeloma, trauma, infection, and—less likely—lymphoma, hemangioma, and underlying lesions such as an aneurysmal bone cyst.

2. Skull, in the parietal bone.

3. Not usually, but remember that marked wedging of an upper lumbar vertebra secondary to hypoplasia is a characteristic finding in the spine, causing angular kyphosis.

4. In vertebra plana, the morphology of the vertebral body was at one time normal.

Reference
Baghaie M, Gillet P, Dondelinger RF, Flandroy P: Vertebra plana: Benign or malignant lesion? Pediatr Radiol 6:431-433, 1996.

Comments
A flattened vertebral body is referred to as a vertebra plana, and the deformity is classically caused by eosinophilic granuloma (EG), although a number of other conditions can produce a flat vertebral morphology. The abnormality is not difficult to identify, and the diagnosis can be relatively straightforward if certain conditions are applied. If the patient is young, consider EG, neuroblastoma metastasis, possibly infection, and possibly trauma; if the patient is elderly, consider metastasis, multiple myeloma, trauma, possibly infection, and possibly lymphoma. If disk space is normal, consider EG, metastasis, multiple myeloma, possibly Paget's disease, and possibly compression fracture. If the end plates are irregular or destroyed, consider infection, tumor, possibly trauma, and possibly Scheuermann's disease. If bone density is decreased, consider trauma, osteoporosis compression fracture, multiple myeloma, metastasis, and possibly osteomalacia. If bone density is increased, consider tumor, trauma, possibly Paget's disease, and possibly hemangioma. If there are multiple vertebral bodies, consider metastasis, multiple myeloma, osteoporosis, and possibly EG. Remember this hint: if you see intravertebral vacuum phenomenon in a collapsed vertebral body, the diagnosis is osteonecrosis (Kümmell's disease).

Myositis Ossificans

1. Myositis ossificans, neoplasm (osteosarcoma, osteochondrosarcoma, chondrosarcoma), and—much less likely—infection.

2. Proliferation of fibroblasts and myofibroblasts and minimal osteoid in a prominent myxoid stroma.

3. Fifty percent of lesions have an association with or are adherent to the periosteum, evoking a periosteal reaction in about 40% in this group.

4. Yes, there would be intense enhancement acutely.

Reference
Yu JS: MR imaging of soft tissue trauma. Emergency Radiol 3:181-194, 1996.

Comments
Myositis ossificans is a benign process, characterized by the formation of an ossifying soft-tissue mass, that occurs in skeletal muscle. The pathogenesis of myositis ossificans is unknown, but it is associated with trauma, burns, and immobilization. Eighty percent of cases involve the large muscles of the extremities, but locations about the scapula, posterior part of the neck, thorax, abdominal wall, and hip have been described. Pain, swelling, and diminished range of motion are common clinical symptoms. As the lesion matures, deposition of cartilage and osteoid takes place, with ossification of the periphery of the lesion. Restriction of motion and pain may sometimes persist for years.

The radiographic findings parallel the histologic pattern of maturation. Initially, the radiographic image is that of soft-tissue swelling (as shown on the CT). Note that high-attenuation blood was present initially as well, because the injury was the result of trauma. After 3 weeks, evidence of maturation may become apparent, with floccular calcifications seen in the periphery of the lesion. At 6 to 8 weeks, lamellar bone with a well-defined cortex surrounds a central radiolucent area (as shown on the radiograph). CT is capable of demonstrating faint mineralization at an early time. In mature lesions, dense peripheral ossification is characteristic and is often associated with a radiolucent zone separating the lesion from the underlying cortex. The magnetic resonance imaging features of myositis ossificans also depend on the stage of the lesion. Acute lesions are isointense to muscle on T1W images. On T2W images, the signal intensity is higher than that of fat, probably related to the cellular areas of proliferating fibroblasts and myofibroblasts. The margins may appear heterogeneous owing to peripheral edema. Subacute lesions demonstrate a border of low signal intensity surrounding the lesion, corresponding to sites of ossification. The center of the lesion may be isointense or slightly higher in signal intensity compared with muscle on T1W images, reflecting areas of fatty infiltration. Fluid-fluid levels and adjacent bone marrow edema may occasionally be present.

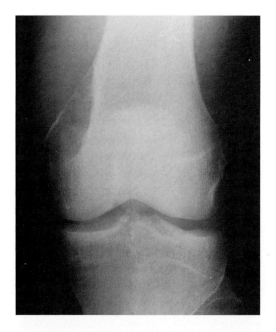
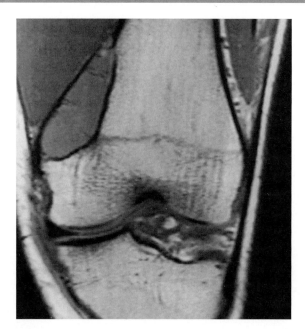

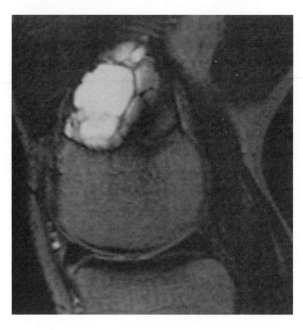

1. What entities would you include in your differential?

2. When present, are fluid-fluid levels specific for an aneurysmal bone cyst?

3. List several malignant tumors that can cause expansile bony metastasis.

4. An aneurysmal bone cyst (ABC) may arise de novo or from a pre-existing lesion. List some of these lesions.

Aneurysmal Bone Cyst

1. ABC, hemorrhagic cyst, and telangiectatic osteogenic sarcoma.

2. No, they can occur in a number of lesions, including giant cell tumor, chondroblastoma, and telangiectatic osteosarcoma, to name a few.

3. Kidney, thyroid, plasmacytoma, malignant fibrous histiocytoma, and—less commonly—melanoma, lung tumor, breast tumor, and pheochromocytoma.

4. Giant cell tumor, osteoblastoma, chondroblastoma, fibrous dysplasia, chondromyxoid fibroma.

Reference

Kransdorf MJ, Sweet DE: Aneurysmal bone cyst: Concept, controversy, clinical presentation, and imaging. AJR Am J Roentgenol 164:573-580, 1995.

Comments

An ABC is an expansile lesion of bone that contains numerous interconnected cavernous cysts that are filled with blood. These cavities, which may have an endothelial lining and numerous multinucleated giant cells, are separated by septations that may show thin bone formation. The majority of ABCs are observed in patients younger than 20 years. The most common symptom is mild, local pain of several months' duration. A pathologic fracture is an uncommon early manifestation of this condition. The long bones, particularly the femur, and the spine are common areas involved, but the flat bones of the pelvis may be affected also. Radiographically, an ABC has an expansile, "bubbly" appearance and is usually found in the metaphysis of a bone. The cortex often appears extremely thinned so that the cortical definition may become inconspicuous on conventional radiographs. At the edges of the lesion, the periosteum may appear elevated and mimic Codman's triangle. Both these radiographic findings may be confused with a malignant process with cortical disruption. Computed tomography and magnetic resonance imaging are useful imaging techniques for further evaluating this lesion. The detection of fluid-fluid levels, representing layering of the blood products within the cavities of an ABC, are typical of this lesion but have been described in other lesions as well.

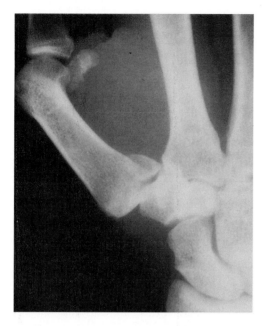

1. How should you report this fracture?

2. What is the treatment of choice?

3. Closed reduction of this fracture may have several complications. Name two.

4. What makes this fracture unstable?

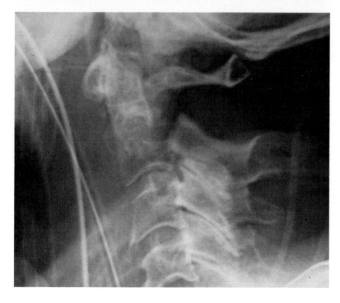

1. What is the diagnosis?

2. What is the Effendi classification?

3. What does anterior displacement of C2 on C3 indicate? Is it unstable?

4. Reportedly, what percentage of people present with neurologic deficits?

Bennett's Fracture

1. Identify the number of fragments, the metacarpal bone displacement, the size and position of the volar fragment, and the fracture gaps that exceed 3 mm.

2. Cast fixation for 6 weeks with or without percutaneous pinning of the basilar fragment.

3. Loss of reduction and pressure necrosis of the skin from cast pressure.

4. Action of the abductor pollicis longus muscle produces distraction, but the pull of the adductor pollicis longus and flexor pollicis brevis, by their more distal attachment, augments the displacement.

Reference

Breen TF, Gelberman RH, Jupiter JB: Intraarticular fractures of the basilar joint of the thumb. Hand Clin 4:491–501, 1988.

Comments

Fracture of the first metacarpal bone is the second most frequent fracture of metacarpal bone after fracture of the fifth metacarpal. Nearly 80% of fractures of this bone involve the base. Basilar fractures can be divided into four types: epibasal, Bennett's, Rolando's, and comminuted. Epibasal fractures are extra-articular fractures through the first metacarpal base and can be transversely or obliquely oriented. Comminuted fractures result in numerous bone fragments and frequently have more than one intra-articular fracture extension. Bennett's fracture is defined as an intra-articular two-part fracture of the base of the first metacarpal. It is the most common thumb fracture, accounting for about one third of all fractures of the first metacarpal bone. Rolando's fracture is a similar fracture, but it produces a three-part fracture. When evaluating radiographs of the first metacarpal, recall the anatomy of the first carpometacarpal joint. The volar oblique ligament, which is intracapsular in location, is the most important stabilizer of this joint. It inserts on the ulnar articular margin of the medial volar beak of the first metacarpal base. When Bennett's or Rolando's fracture occurs, the medial volar beak remains attached to this ligament while the rest of the metacarpal base becomes displaced radially owing to the pull of the abductor pollicis muscle.

Hangman's Fracture

1. Hangman's fracture.

2. Classification of hangman's fractures based on the relationship of C2 on C3.

3. Damage to the C2 disk and anterior longitudinal ligament. Yes.

4. Ten percent.

Reference

Effendi B, Roy D, Cornish B, et al: Fractures of the ring of the axis. J Bone Joint Surg Br 63:319–327, 1981.

Comments

Bilateral fracture of the neural arch of C2 is called hangman's fracture. It is usually caused by a hyperextension injury, although flexion-compression and flexion-distraction injuries may occasionally cause this fracture. The vast majority of these fractures are caused by motor vehicle accidents. Because there is no encroachment of the spinal canal, neurologic deficits are uncommon in this injury and are generally not permanent. Hangman's fractures have been classified by Effendi et al into three types, based on the relationship of C2 on C3. In type 1 fractures, there is no forward displacement of C2 on C3, and the fractures involve only the posterior elements. In type 2 fractures, there is anterior displacement of C2 on C3. In type 3 fractures, there is anterior displacement of both anterior and posterior fragments. Generally, both type 2 and type 3 require halo immobilization. It is important to realize that other fractures of the cervical spine are common in patients with a hangman's fracture. Fractures of the C1 arch occur in 15% of cases, fractures of the body of C2 (as in this patient) occur in another 15% of cases, and 10% of patients also have a fracture in the thoracic spine.

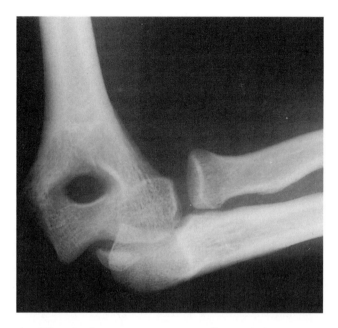
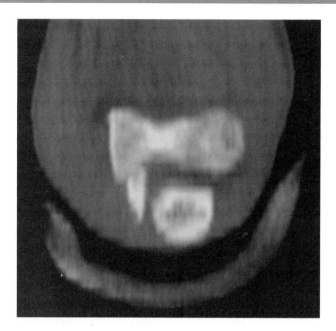

1. What is the most common elbow dislocation? How do most posterior elbow dislocations occur?
2. What fractures are commonly associated with elbow dislocations? How often do they occur?
3. What complication did you notice in this patient? What happened during reduction?
4. What anatomic relationship allows this injury to occur?

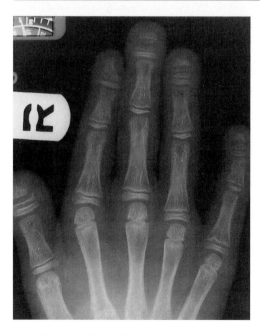
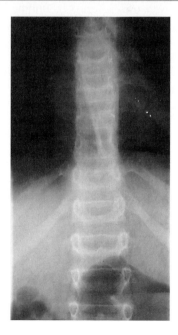

1. What is the differential diagnosis list for acro-osteolysis?
2. What neoplasm is associated with exposure to polyvinyl chloride?
3. What neuropathic disorder do acro-osteolysis and calcification of digital nerves characterize?
4. In a skeletally immature person, what part of the distal phalanx is most vulnerable to thermal injuries?

Avulsion of the Medial Epicondylar Ossification Center

1. Posterior. Fall on an outstretched hand.

2. Fractures of the coronoid process, humeral epicondyles, and radial head. Twenty-five percent of cases.

3. Avulsion of the medial epicondylar ossification center. It became entrapped in the joint.

4. The ulnar collateral ligament and the flexor pronator tendon attach to the undersurface of the medial epicondyle.

Reference

Woods GW, Tullos HS: Elbow instability and medial epicondyle fractures. Am J Sports Med 5:23-30, 1977.

Comments

Dislocation of the elbow is a relatively common injury in children. Dislocations may involve only the radius, only the ulna, or both bones. Posterior dislocations account for 80% to 90% of elbow dislocations. In children, avulsion of the medial epicondylar ossification center and entrapment into the joint during reduction are important complications. Postreduction radiographs are necessary to ensure that anatomic alignment has been restored. To be able to recognize a growth plate injury, recall the pattern of ossification about the elbow. The acronym CRITOE gets you in the ballpark: *c*apitulum (year 1); *r*adial head (years 3 to 6); *i*nternal or medial epicondyle (years 5 to 7); *t*rochlea (years 9 and 10); *o*lecranon (years 6 to 10); and *e*xternal or lateral epicondyle (years 9 to 13). Absence of a medial epicondyle in a patient who has ossification of the trochlear or lateral epicondylar ossification centers should arouse your suspicion for an avulsion. The treatment of an avulsed medial epicondylar ossification center is surgical realignment, immobilization for a short duration, and early motion through a protected arc to avoid a flexion contracture. When a fracture is present, it is critical to determine that a fracture fragment will not impede motion. Computed tomography is often required to evaluate the joint space, and magnetic resonance imaging adds valuable information about ligamentous disruption.

Acro-osteolysis (Hajdu-Cheney Syndrome)

1. Diffuse pattern: collagen vascular disease and vasculitis, Raynaud's disease, neuropathic disease, thermal injuries, hyperparathyroidism, trauma, epidermolysis bullosa, abnormal stresses, psoriasis, frostbite, sarcoid, hypertrophic osteoarthropathy, pyknodysostosis. Bandlike resorption: polyvinyl chloride exposure and Hajdu-Cheney syndrome.

2. Angiosarcoma of the liver.

3. Leprosy (Hansen's disease).

4. The growth plate.

References

Destouet JM, Murphy WA: Acquired acroosteolysis and acronecrosis. Arthritis Rheum 26:1150-1154, 1983.

Weleber RG, Beals RK: The Hajdu-Cheney syndrome. Report of two cases and review of the literature. J Pediatr 88:243-249, 1976.

Comments

Destruction or resorption of the distal phalanges of the hand describes acro-osteolysis, and this process is associated with numerous etiologies. In many situations, it is impossible to determine the precise cause of the bone lysis when one is asked to rely exclusively on radiographs of the hands. It is important to observe findings elsewhere in the skeleton and to make use of relevant clinical history to render a more specific diagnosis. The pattern of bone lysis is helpful in narrowing the diagnostic considerations, however. There are two patterns of acro-osteolysis in adults. One pattern preferentially involves the tufts of the terminal phalanges, whereas the other pattern creates a band of osteolysis in the midportion of these bones. The differential diagnosis for bandlike resorption is narrower than that for the diffuse pattern of lysis. Bandlike resorption should bring to mind polyvinyl chloride toxicity, Hajdu-Cheney syndrome, and—occasionally—hyperparathyroidism, collagen vascular diseases, and abnormal stresses. In the latter three situations, more classic tufted resorption typically coexists. This patient had Hajdu-Cheney syndrome. The key to the diagnosis was based on two important observations. The first clue was a diffuse pattern of bandlike resorption. The second clue was generalized osteoporosis with vertebral body compression fractures.

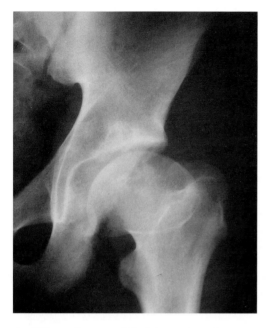
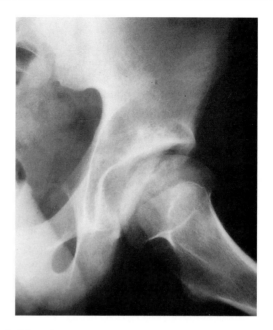

1. What disease did this patient have as a child?
2. What are the stages of this disease?
3. Who is likely to develop secondary osteoarthritis?
4. What is meant by trochanteric overgrowth? Does the patient have this?

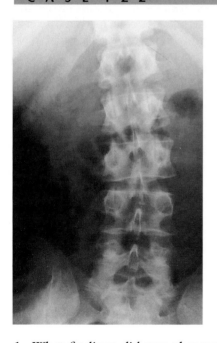
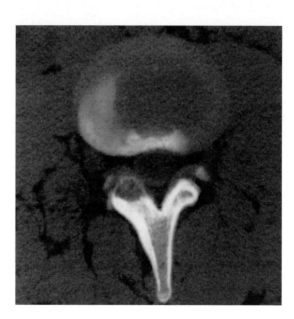

1. What findings did you observe in the spine?
2. Describe a "double density" sign on a bone scan.
3. What is the histology of the nidus of this neoplasm?
4. What is the characteristic appearance of this lesion when it involves a carpal or tarsal bone?

C A S E 1 2 1

Legg-Calvé-Perthes Disease

1. Legg-Calvé-Perthes disease.

2. The avascular phase is characterized by ischemia. The revascularization phase is represented by the ingrowth of highly vascular fibrous tissue and the formation of new bone. The reparative phase is characterized by remodeling of the femoral head.

3. Patients who develop Legg-Calvé-Perthes disease after age 9 years. There is minimal potential for the acetabulum to remodel to the deformed femoral head, in contradistinction to the potential for younger patients.

4. Disproportionately larger greater trochanter owing to a shortened femoral neck. Yes.

Reference

Wall EJ: Legg-Calvé-Perthes' disease. Curr Opin Pediatr 11:76–79, 1999.

Comments

Legg-Calvé-Perthes disease is a self-limiting disorder characterized by necrosis of the ossification center of the femoral capital epiphysis. It occurs at a peak age of 4 to 6 years and has a strong male predilection with a male-to-female ratio of 4:1. The most common initial manifestation is a painful hip that causes a limp. Although an etiology has not yet been determined, most experts believe that this process is secondary to a loss of circulation of the femoral capital epiphysis, with subsequent development of necrosis of the femoral head. In this case, one needs to ask "When did the insult occur?" because the age of onset correlates with the degree of deformity of the femoral head. Patients who present at younger than 5 years have less femoral head deformation than do patients who suffer the disease later in life. The earliest changes include slight lateral displacement of the femur and widening of the hip joint space. Often, the epiphysis (ossification center) is smaller than the normal contralateral side. As the disease progresses, subchondral fractures occur, which flatten the femoral head contour. With reossification and remodeling of the femoral head, a characteristic "mushroom-shaped" head develops on a short, thick, femoral neck (coxa magna deformity), as seen in this patient. A widened joint space usually persists into adulthood.

C A S E 1 2 2

Osteoid Osteoma

1. Dense L3 lamina and thickened cortex in the L3 spinous process with scoliosis, concave toward the side of the lesion.

2. A small focal area of intense radionuclide uptake superimposed on a larger region of less intense activity, typical of an osteoid osteoma.

3. Bone in various stages of maturation within a highly vascular connective tissue stroma that contains numerous dilated capillaries.

4. Round, well-circumscribed, calcified lesion surrounded by a lucent rim with no reactive sclerosis.

Reference

Shankman S, Desai P, Beltran J: Subperiosteal osteoid osteoma: Radiographic and pathologic manifestations. Skeletal Radiol 26:457–462, 1997.

Comments

Osteoid osteoma is a tumor that affects young people; 90% of cases occur in people younger than 25 years. There is a predilection for males by a male-to-female ratio of 3:1. Pain is the hallmark of this benign lesion, which tends to be worse at night and ameliorated by small doses of aspirin. Initially, the pain is mild and transient, but it then becomes severe and persistent. Soft-tissue swelling and tenderness may accompany the pain when it is severe. The nidus of an osteoid osteoma, the essential lesion of this tumor, is usually small, measuring less than 1 cm in diameter. This nidus may eventually calcify, but it is initially devoid of calcium. Reactive sclerosis, such as cortical thickening and periostitis, is a dominant secondary feature of this lesion. The degree of reactive bone is influenced by the location of the nidus. An intracapsular osteoid osteoma, for example, elicits less reactive sclerosis than does a subperiosteal lesion in the shaft of the femur.

In the long bone and spine, computed tomography is essential in demonstrating the location of the radiolucent nidus, which is often obscured by reactive bone on radiographs. The superficial location is helpful in differentiating an osteoid osteoma from a longitudinal stress fracture in the long bones. Reactive sclerosis may be more difficult to identify when the osteoid osteoma involves the spine. Look for a scoliotic curvature, which identifies the side of the lesion (concavity of the curve), but take notice that there is no rotatory component, a typical finding in patients with idiopathic scoliosis. Notable observations include a dense pedicle, lamina, transverse process, or spinous process.

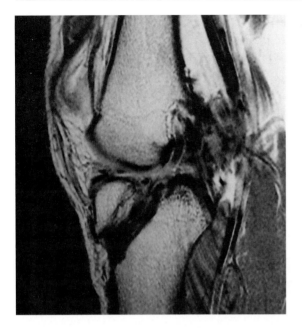 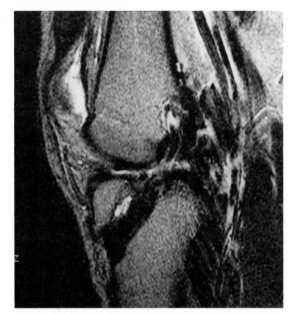

1. What surgery did this patient have? What is the status of the graft?
2. What is the most common cause of graft impingement?
3. At what knee position is graft impingement most evident? Is this obvious to the arthroscopist?
4. What injury mechanisms can cause rupture of a reconstructed anterior cruciate ligament (ACL)?

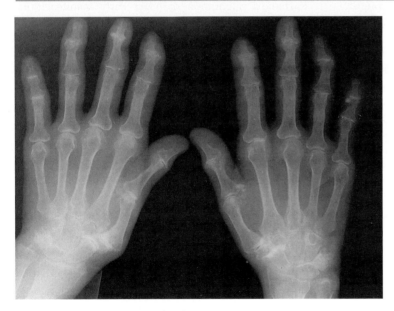

1. What is the differential diagnosis?
2. What conditions cause erosions at the distal interphalangeal (DIP) and proximal interphalangeal (PIP) joints?
3. What is CREST syndrome?
4. List the target organs in patients with this disease.

ACL Graft Tear

1. ACL reconstruction. Torn.

2. The tibial tunnel is positioned too far anteriorly on the tibia.

3. Most evident in the terminal 5 to 10 degrees of extension. No.

4. The same mechanisms that would rupture a native ACL.

Reference

Recht MP, Piraino DW, Applegate G, et al: Complications after anterior cruciate ligament reconstruction: Radiographic and MR findings. AJR Am J Roentgenol 167:705–710, 1996.

Comments

There are different methods for reconstructing a torn ACL ligament, but an intra-articular reconstruction using a patellar tendon graft is currently the preferred technique. In this surgical procedure, the central third of the patellar tendon is resected with bone plugs at each end, and this graft is secured in bone tunnels in the posterolateral femur and anterior tibia by interference screws. Proper positioning of the bone tunnels is important in maintaining isometry of the graft and, more importantly, in preventing graft impingement. On a lateral radiograph, the femoral tunnel should be positioned at the intersection of Blumensaat's line (the intercondylar roof) and a line representing the posterior femoral cortex. The position of the tibial tunnel should be entirely posterior and parallel to the tibial intersection of Blumensaat's line when the knee is in full extension. An ACL graft may become impinged on either the sidewall or the roof of the intercondylar notch, and this complication most commonly occurs when the tibial tunnel is placed too anteriorly on the tibia. On magnetic resonance imaging, increased signal intensity occurs at the point of impingement, and when it is extensive, the edema may obscure visualization of any intact fibers. An impinged ACL graft is at risk for rupture. On magnetic resonance imaging, a complete rupture appears as an absence of intact fibers in the intercondylar notch associated with high signal intensity on T2W images, indicating edema.

Scleroderma

1. Scleroderma, dermatomyositis, Ehlers-Danlos disease, and hyperparathyroidism.

2. Psoriasis, erosive osteoarthritis, multicentric reticulohistiocytosis, gout, scleroderma, and rheumatoid arthritis.

3. Calcinosis, Raynaud's phenomenon, esophageal abnormalities, sclerodactyly, and telangiectasia.

4. The skin, gastrointestinal tract, lungs, kidneys, heart, and structures of the musculoskeletal system.

Reference

Gold RH, Bassett LW, Seeger LL: The other arthritides. Roentgenologic features of osteoarthritis, erosive osteoarthritis, ankylosing spondylitis, psoriatic arthritis, Reiter's disease, multicentric reticulohistiocytosis, and progressive systemic sclerosis. Radiol Clin North Am 26:1195–1212, 1988.

Comments

Scleroderma is an uncommon disorder of unknown etiology that is characterized by small vessel disease and fibrosis in several organ systems. Scleroderma affects females more frequently than males by a female-to-male ratio of 3:1. The disorder becomes clinically evident by the third to fifth decade of life. A common presentation is Raynaud's phenomenon; other early manifestations include thickening of the skin and edema of the extremities. Pain and stiffness involving the small joints of the hands and knees and dysphagia are also typical presenting complaints. With progression of the disease, skin changes in the fingers, face, and feet become predominant features, appearing taut, shiny, and atrophic. The soft tissues of the distal fingers become tapered, and ulcerated subcutaneous calcific deposits develop in more extensive disease.

Radiographically, abnormalities of the hands are characterized by resorption of the soft tissues, often producing a conical shape to the ends of the digits, subcutaneous calcifications, and acro-osteolysis. Nearly 75% of patients with calcinosis demonstrate calcific deposits in the hands (notice the thumb, fifth finger, and wrist of right hand). These calcifications may occur in the subcutaneous tissues or in the joint capsule. Erosions similar to those in rheumatoid arthritis are common and may occur in 40% to 80% of patients affected. But a distinctive feature of these erosions is their predilection for the PIP and DIP joints. Remember that severe resorption of the first carpometacarpal joint with radial subluxation of the first metacarpal bone is nearly pathognomonic of scleroderma (seen in both hands in this patient).

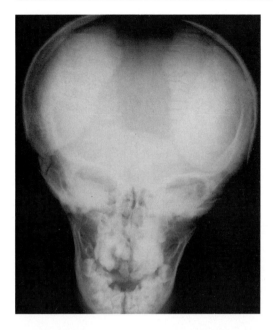
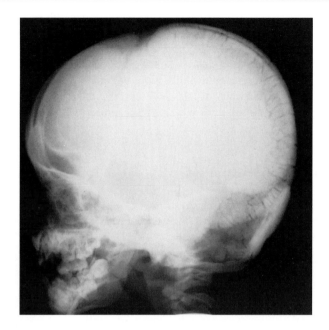

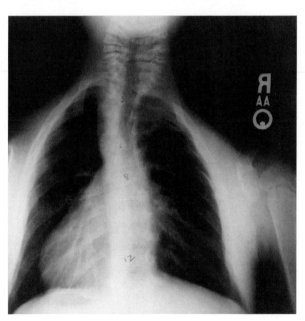

1. What is your diagnosis?
2. What are the major findings in the skull? Is there a differential consideration based on these findings?
3. What percentage of patients have completely absent clavicles?
4. How is this condition transmitted? What is the life expectancy?

Cleidocranial Dysplasia

1. Cleidocranial dysplasia.

2. Wormian bones, basilar invagination, delayed closure of anterior fontanel, enlarged skull with widened sutures, and supernumerary teeth. Differential may include pyknodysostosis and osteogenesis imperfecta.

3. Ten percent.

4. Autosomal dominant. Normal.

Reference

Jarvis JL, Keats TE: Cleidocranial dysostosis. The review of 40 cases. AJR Am J Roentgenol 121:5–16, 1974.

Comments

This congenital condition, also known as cleidocranial dysostosis, is caused by a defect in ossification. A faulty anlage for intramembranous bone formation, particularly of the clavicle and calvarium, is the suspected defect. Patients have a large head with a disproportionately small face, narrow chest, and drooping shoulders. The shoulders often have unusual mobility, so that some patients can voluntarily approximate their shoulders to the point of touching anteriorly. Radiographically, the defective ossification of the skull produces wide sutures, wormian bones, and enlargement of the foramen magnum. The facial bones are hypoplastic, as are the paranasal sinuses. The most common defect is absence of the distal clavicles. Fragmentation and failure to fuse are also common clavicular features. In about 10% of cases, the entire clavicle is absent. In the pelvis, the most frequent finding is a wide pubic symphysis, although defective ossification of the ischium and hypoplasia of the ilium are not uncommon. Occasionally, the radius and femoral neck may be hypoplastic or absent. In the hands, extranumerary ossification centers have been reported, resulting in elongation of the second metacarpal bone.

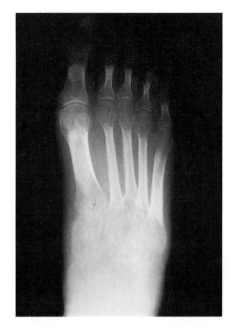 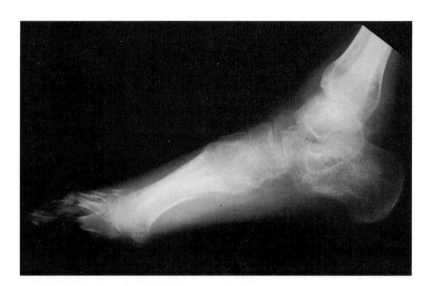

1. What are the radiographic findings, and what is the main diagnostic consideration?
2. List the neoplasms that may be associated with this condition.
3. What are the characteristic clinical features of this disorder?
4. Five types of bone resorption are associated with this syndrome. List them.

Reflex Sympathetic Dystrophy

1. Diffuse periarticular osteopenia and soft-tissue swelling. Reflex sympathetic dystrophy (RSD).

2. Malignant tumors of the brain, lung, ovary, breast, pancreas, and bladder.

3. Stiffness, pain, tenderness, and weakness associated with swelling, hyperesthesia, and vasomotor changes.

4. Cancellous or trabecular resorption in the metaphysis; subperiosteal resorption, similar to hyperparathyroidism; intracortical resorption, producing tunneling; endosteal resorption, causing scalloping and widening of medullary canal; and subchondral and juxta-articular erosion, simulating a primary arthritis.

Reference

Resnick D, Niwayama G: Osteoporosis. In Resnick D (ed): Diagnosis of Bone and Joint Disorders, 3rd ed. Philadelphia, WB Saunders, 1995, pp 1797–1802.

Comments

RSD, also known as Sudeck's atrophy, is a painful condition most commonly caused by trauma. Myocardial infarction, hemiplegia, cerebrovascular accident, disk herniation, surgery, infection, vasculitis, and neoplasms may also elicit this disorder. Although the pathogenesis of RSD is not clear, the most widely accepted theory is that an injury or lesion produces painful impulses that are sent to the spinal cord through afferent pathways, establishing a series of reflexes. These reflexes stimulate efferent pathways that travel to the peripheral nerves, producing the findings associated with this condition. There are data that support the suggestion that RSD is related to overactivity of the sympathetic nervous system. One fourth to one half of cases are bilateral, although RSD tends to affect one side more severely than the other.

The radiographic findings of this condition are characteristic. Soft-tissue swelling and regional osteoporosis are prominent features. Resorption of cancellous or trabecular bone in the metaphyseal region leads to periarticular osteoporosis. Although this finding may also occur in synovial inflammatory arthropathies, the absence of joint space loss and erosions is a notable observation. Bone scintigraphy demonstrates increased radionuclide uptake in an articular distribution caused by increased vascularity of the synovial membrane and bones.

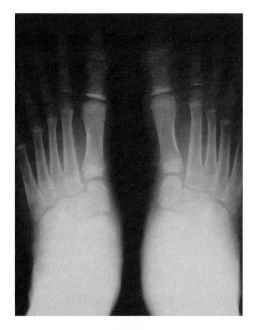
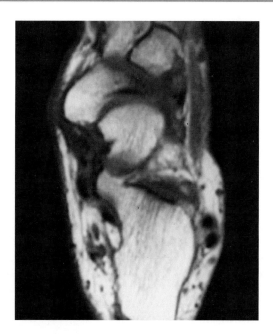

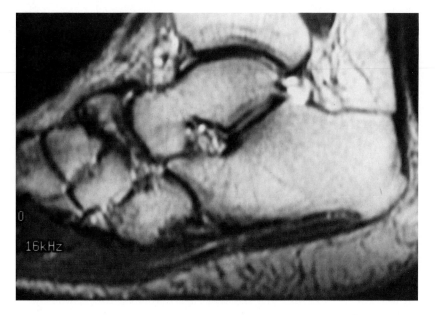

1. Magnetic resonance imaging (MRI) was performed 6 years after the radiograph. What is the most likely diagnosis?

2. Could this be a stress fracture?

3. What are the criteria for Köhler's disease?

4. What would a bone scan show in a patient with acute Köhler's disease?

Osteochondrosis of the Tarsal Navicular (Köhler's Disease)

1. Idiopathic osteonecrosis of the tarsal navicular (Köhler's disease).

2. No, most navicular stress fractures are vertically oriented in the sagittal plane, involve the medial or middle portions of the bone, and are not associated with collapse.

3. There are three criteria: (1) changes are identified in a previously normal navicular bone, (2) findings are compatible with osteonecrosis, and (3) it affects children.

4. Diminished uptake of the radionuclide agent during the early phase of the disease and increased uptake during revascularization.

Reference

Haller J, Sartoris DJ, Resnick D, et al: Spontaneous osteonecrosis of the tarsal navicular in adults: Imaging findings. AJR Am J Roentgenol 151:355–358, 1988.

Comments

Köhler's disease, idiopathic osteonecrosis of the tarsal navicular, is a rare condition that affects young children, commonly those between the ages of 3 and 7 years. Boys are four times more frequently affected than are girls. Most cases involve one foot, although as many as 25% of cases are bilateral. Clinically, pain, tenderness, swelling, and limited range of motion are common manifestations, and about one third of patients recall a history of trauma. Some experts have hypothesized that compression of the ossification centers of the navicular at a critical phase of growth may result in altered ossification, in part from ischemia caused by occlusion of vessels in the spongiosa of the bone. The radiographic features of Köhler's disease are fragmentation and increased density in the ossification centers of the tarsal navicular bone, which produce a flattened appearance. The morphology of the bone may return to normal, or the deformity may persist throughout a patient's life. The self-limited and reversible nature of the process in certain patients has led to the speculation that in some people, Köhler's disease actually represents a variation in the ossification of the tarsal bone.

The main differential is Mueller-Weiss disease (spontaneous osteonecrosis of the navicular in adults), which is likely caused by chronic stress from an abnormal plantar arch and secondary osteonecrosis and by post-traumatic osteonecrosis. The radiographic findings are similar with decreased tarsal size, a comma-shaped configuration, increased radiodensity, fragmentation, and medial or medial and dorsal osseous protrusion.

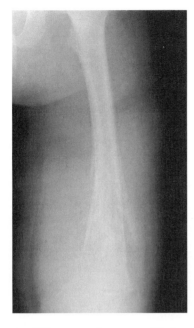 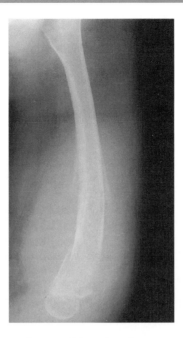

1. What are the most likely diagnostic considerations?

2. In patients diagnosed with neuroblastoma, what is the cause of widened cranial sutures?

3. What substance may be found in the urine of patients with neuroblastoma?

4. What is the histologic differential diagnosis for round cell tumors?

Neuroblastoma Metastasis

1. Neuroblastoma metastasis, leukemia, lymphoma, infection, and eosinophilic granuloma.

2. Increased intracranial pressure from leptomeningeal metastases.

3. Vanillylmandelic acid.

4. Myeloma, lymphoma, Ewing's sarcoma, neuroblastoma, rhabdomyosarcoma, small cell carcinoma, and primitive neuroectodermal tumor.

Reference

Roberts JL, Magid D, Miller NR, et al: Case report 493: Neuroblastoma of the left ilium with disseminated bony metastasis. Skeletal Radiol 17:375–377, 1988.

Comments

The radiographic findings in this patient clearly indicate an aggressive lesion, but otherwise the findings are rather nonspecific. Permeative bone destruction is evident in the distal femur, with periosteal new bone formation outlining the margins of a large soft-tissue mass involving the metaphysis of the bone. A pathologic fracture has occurred just above growth plate. The differential diagnosis includes metastasis (medulloblastoma, rhabdomyosarcoma, retinoblastoma, Wilms' tumor), leukemia, lymphoma, Ewing's sarcoma, osteogenic sarcoma, eosinophilic granuloma, and infection. The most distinctive feature in this patient is his age, which is 2 years. In this particular case, the diagnosis of metastatic neuroblastoma is the best diagnosis, and Ewing's sarcoma, infection, and leukemia are secondary considerations.

Neuroblastoma is a common childhood neoplasm arising in the adrenal medulla; it is known for its aggressive behavior, widespread metastases, and rapid growth. Nearly 75% of cases occur in patients younger than 4 years, and more than 90% occur in patients younger than 8 years. In most situations, the patient already has skeletal metastases at the time of diagnosis. Permeative bone destruction is characteristic, although sclerosis may occur with healing or as a late manifestation of the disease. Horizontal radiolucent zones in the metaphysis may resemble those seen in leukemic patients. Occasionally, patients may present with vertebra plana, leading to spinal cord compression from an adjacent soft-tissue mass, or a pathologic fracture of a long bone.

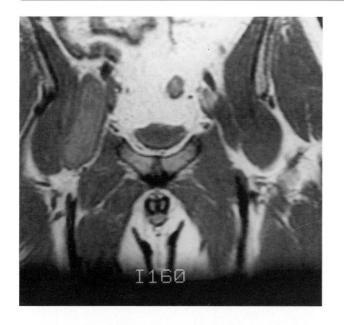
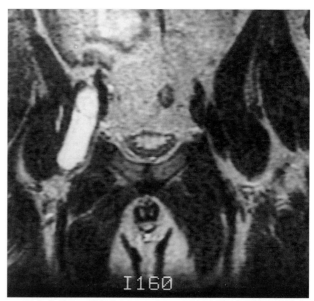
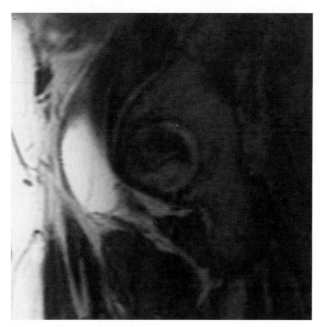

1. Can the iliopsoas bursa communicate with the hip joint? Where?
2. What conditions can cause distention of the iliopsoas bursa?
3. What is "snapping iliopsoas tendon" syndrome?
4. What does an avulsion of the lesser trochanter suggest?

Iliopsoas Bursitis

1. Yes. Between the iliofemoral and pubofemoral ligaments.

2. Conditions that cause synovitis such as osteoarthritis, rheumatoid arthritis, pigmented villonodular synovitis, and synovial chondromatosis.

3. Overuse syndrome characterized by inflammation caused by rubbing of the iliopsoas tendon over the iliopectineal eminence on the pubis.

4. Metastasis.

Reference

Pritchard RS, Shah HR, Nelson CL, Ritzrandolph RL: MR and CT appearance of iliopsoas bursal distension secondary to diseased hips. J Comp Assist Tomogr 14:797–808, 1990.

Comments

The iliopsoas bursa is the largest bursa around the hip joint and is present in 98% of people. It is located anterior to the joint capsule in close proximity to the iliopsoas muscle. The bursa communicates with the hip joint through a space between the iliofemoral and pubofemoral ligaments in 15% of normal hips. Fluid may accumulate within the iliopsoas bursa, creating a mass in the inguinal region of the hip, which can sometimes compress the femoral vein, bladder, or colon. Synovitis from a number of arthritic processes may cause distention of the bursa with fluid. Distention of this space causes pain that is easily confused with other conditions. Magnetic resonance imaging has proved to be an important diagnostic technique for diagnosing iliopsoas bursitis and pathology related to the iliopsoas tendon. T2W images demonstrate a fluid-containing structure, depicted by high signal intensity, adjacent to the iliopsoas tendon in a characteristic location anterior to the hip joint.

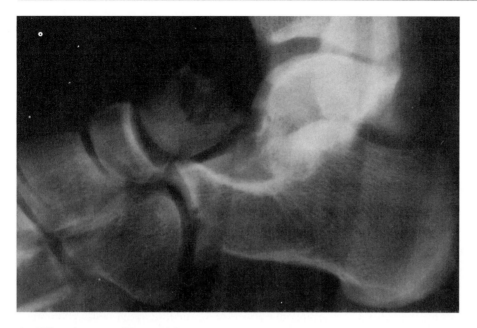

1. What is your diagnosis?

2. Describe the mechanism of injury.

3. What is the Hawkins sign, and what does it mean?

4. In the Hawkins classification, what is the risk of developing avascular necrosis (AVN) for each classification?

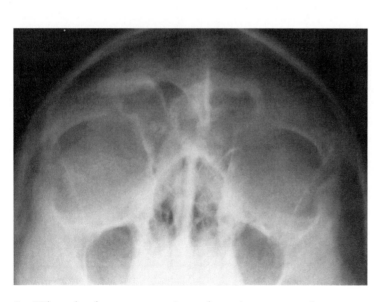 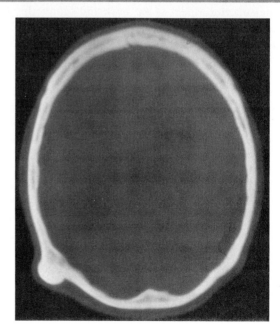

1. What do these two patients have in common?

2. Describe Gardner's syndrome.

3. Is there a cartilage cap associated with this lesion?

4. How does this lesion differ from a bone island?

Talar Neck Fracture

1. Fractures of the talar neck and anterior process of the calcaneus.

2. Abrupt dorsiflexion of the forefoot, probably from a motor vehicle accident or a fall.

3. Subchondral lucidity in the talar dome from disuse osteoporosis, which indicates an intact vascular supply.

4. AVN occurs in less than 5% of type 1 fractures, 33% of type 2 fractures, and nearly all of type 3 fractures.

Reference

Canale ST, Kelley FB: Fractures of the neck and the talus. J Bone Joint Surg Am 60:143-156, 1978.

Comments

Fractures of the talar neck are uncommon in adults and rare in children, but this injury accounts for the second most frequent type of fracture involving the talus. It is most often associated with motor vehicle accidents and falls, but occasionally a direct impaction to the dorsum of the foot may cause this fracture. When evaluating a talar neck fracture, recall the vascular supply to this bone. The main blood supply enters the talus through the tarsal tunnel as a branch of the posterior tibial artery. It supplies the inferior neck and most of the body. The dorsalis pedis artery and its branches enter the superior aspect of the neck and supply the dorsum of the neck and head regions. The peroneal artery supplies a portion of the lateral talus.

The Hawkins classification prognosticates the risk of developing AVN in patients who have fractures of the talus. Type 1 fractures are nondisplaced and bisect the subtalar joint between the middle and posterior facets. The vascular supply is generally preserved. Type 2 fractures are displaced with subluxation or dislocation of the subtalar joint, disrupting two (occasionally three) of the vascular supplies. Type 3 fractures are displaced with dislocation of the body from both the tibiotalar and subtalar joints, disrupting all three vascular supplies. Type 4 fractures have an associated talonavicular subluxation or dislocation. Eighty percent of talar neck fractures are type 2 or 3 fractures. The incidence of type 1 fractures is about 15%, and type 4 fractures make up the remaining 5%.

Skull Osteoma

1. Both have an osteoma.

2. Adenomatous polyposis of the colon, dental lesions, soft-tissue tumors, and osteomas.

3. No.

4. A bone island is contained within the medullary cavity of a bone.

Reference

Earwaker J: Paranasal sinus osteomas: A review of 46 cases. Skeletal Radiol 22:417-423, 1993.

Comments

An osteoma is a masslike protrusion of extremely dense bone arising from the periosteum. It is caused by exaggerated intramembranous bone formation. Histologically, these lesions are composed of wide, irregularly arranged trabeculae of mature bone with prominent osteoid seams and a sparse amount of tissue between the trabeculation. A periosteal membrane covers the outer surface of the osteoma. Most lesions are detected in middle-aged patients, although osteomas can affect people of any age. The common locations affected are the skull, facial bones, and tubular bones. There is high frequency of osteoma in the frontal sinus. When it affects the calvarium, it can arise from either skull table, although the outer table is much more commonly affected. Symptoms are usually related to encroachment of the protruding mass into a space, such as the sinuses, orbits, cranial vault, or mouth.

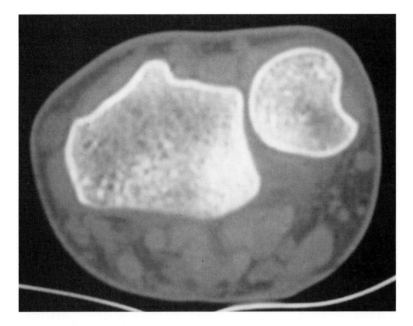

1. Where is the sigmoid notch?
2. How is instability of the distal radioulnar joint (DRUJ) best assessed?
3. What are some causes of joint instability?
4. Define an Essex-Lopresti injury.

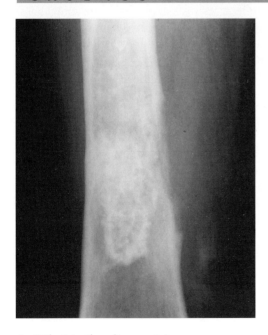

1. What is the diagnosis?
2. Who is at risk for developing this complication?
3. What is the histology of the neoplasms?
4. Is this lesion common? When does this complication occur?

Dorsal Ulnar Instability

1. On the medial surface of the radius where the ulna articulates.

2. By computed tomography (CT) or magnetic resonance imaging (MRI) with full pronation and supination of the wrist.

3. Fracture of the distal radius or ulna, ulnar minus variance, injuries to the triangular fibrocartilage complex.

4. Fracture or fracture-dislocation of the radial head associated with disruption of the interosseous membrane between the radius and the ulna and with dislocation of the DRUJ.

Reference

Nakamura R, Horii E, Imaeda T, Nakao E: Criteria for diagnosing distal radioulnar joint subluxation by computed tomography. Skeletal Radiol 25:649–653, 1996.

Comments

Dorsal subluxation of the distal ulna is the most common type of instability that affects the DRUJ. This abnormality is caused by a hyperpronation injury to the wrist. Clinically, the distal ulna appears prominent. Radiographically, the abnormality may be evident on frontal radiographs of the wrist. There is widening and, less frequently, overlapping or incongruity of the DRUJ. Volar dislocation of the DRUJ is caused by hypersupination stress to the forearm. Clinically, the patient presents with a forearm maintained in supination. Radiographically, there is palmar displacement of the distal ulna on the lateral view.

Cross-sectional imaging techniques such as CT scanning and MRI are useful for assessment of the DRUJ because they allow direct inspection of the articulation. Assessment of instability should be performed with full pronation and supination of the wrist. Between these positions, the distal radius can actively rotate about 150 degrees around the ulnar head when the elbow is flexed and 190 degrees through passive motion. Maximum contact between the ulnar head and radius occurs when the forearm is in midrotation. There are three different techniques for evaluating the integrity of the DRUJ on CT or MRI (epicenter method, Mino's method, and congruency method). In this case, the ulna is displaced dorsally, resulting in a positive Mino's sign (ulna exceeds dorsal radioulnar line of the radius) and negative congruency (disrupted articular parallelism).

Sarcoma Associated with a Bone Infarct

1. Malignant transformation of a bone infarct.

2. Men in the fifth to seventh decades of life.

3. Malignant fibrous histiocytoma and osteosarcoma.

4. No, it is rare. After many years, there is a long latent period between bone infarction and malignant transformation.

References

Galli SJ, Weintraub HP, Proppe KH: Malignant fibrous histiocytoma and pleomorphic sarcoma in association with medullary bone infarcts. Cancer 41:607–619, 1978.

Mirra JM, Gold RH, Marafiote R: Malignant (fibrous) histiocytoma arising in association with a bone infarct in sickle-cell disease: Coincidence or cause-and-effect? Cancer 39:186–194, 1977.

Comments

The radiographic appearance of a mature bone infarct is distinctive and is seldom a cause for concern. Infarcts are intramedullary lesions that have a characteristic serpentine rim of dense sclerosis surrounding a variably calcified central area. Occasionally, one must differentiate an infarct from an enchondroma, but several observations, including internal or central calcifications and lack of peripheral sclerosis in the latter, are sufficient to avoid confusion between these two entities.

An infarct can undergo two processes that may alter its appearance, and both are rare. Cyst formation occurs most frequently in the humerus, followed by the tibia, femur, ilium, and calcaneus. These cysts may erode the endosteal cortex. Malignant transformation also may alter the appearance of an infarct. The majority of cases involve the femur, tibia, and humerus. The lesions are poorly differentiated, containing fibrous, osteoid, or cartilaginous tissue, and have a poor prognosis. The radiographic diagnosis is not challenging, and this case of a malignant fibrous histiocytoma arising in association with an infarct in the distal femur is fairly typical. There is osseous destruction of the medial cortex, elevation of the periosteum forming Codman's triangles, and a soft-tissue mass at the site of a previous infarct. In some patients, the sarcomatous proliferation may eventually obliterate all evidence of a pre-existent infarct.

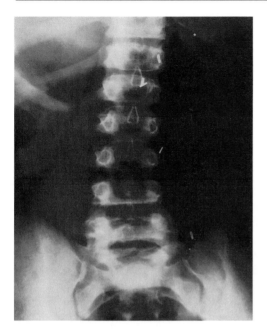 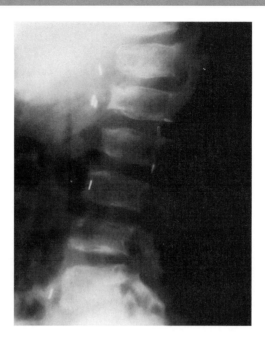

1. Describe the findings.
2. What factors determine the severity of the scoliosis? How soon after treatment would you expect to see skeletal changes?
3. What was the lowest dose used in this case?
4. What would magnetic resonance imaging of this spine show?

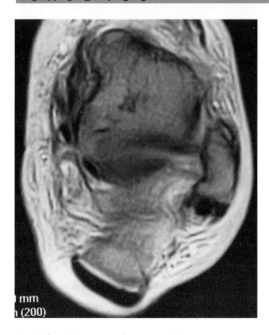

1. What is your diagnosis?
2. Where do most peroneus brevis tendon tears begin?
3. Is it normal to have fluid in either of the peroneal tendon sheaths?
4. What are predisposing factors that contribute to tears of the peroneus brevis tendon?

Radiation-Induced Scoliosis (T11–L5)

1. Scoliosis (mild), hypoplasia of the T11–L5 pedicles on the left, and flattening of the vertebral bodies with scalloping of the end plates.

2. Dose, age, field size. As early as 6 months after treatment.

3. At least 3000 cGy.

4. Decreased hematopoietic marrow and replacement with fatty marrow.

Reference

Makipernaa A, Heikkila JT, Merikanto J, et al: Spinal deformity induced by radiotherapy for solid tumours in childhood: A long-term follow up study. Eur J Pediatr 152:197–200, 1993.

Comments

Radiation therapy is an important facet of medicine and is used for the treatment of a number of pediatric neoplasms. A field irradiated with a sufficient dose can suppress or arrest the growth of bones that are exposed. This consequence of treatment has great significance when the lesion is near or in the spine, such as with renal neoplasm, neuroblastoma, medulloblastoma, ependymoma, and astrocytoma. The key finding in this case is scoliosis. Your job is to determine why the scoliosis is present. There are two types of scoliosis that are related to postradiation changes, lateral flexion curve (as in this case), and rotatory changes (primarily in the posterior elements). The dose is the most important factor in determining the changes in the bone. When the dose is less than 2000 cGy, little change is seen. Between 2000 to 3000 cGy, partial growth arrest may result in a "bone-in-bone" appearance and scoliosis of less than 20 degrees, and beyond 3000 cGy, flattening of the vertebral body, scalloping of the end plates, and growth cessation are pronounced, with scoliosis greater than 20 degrees. The disk spaces maintain a normal height. This patient had been treated with 4500 cGy for a Wilms' tumor involving the left kidney.

Peroneus Brevis Tendon Tear

1. Longitudinal tear of the peroneus brevis tendon.

2. Either just distal to the fibular tip or beyond the inferior extensor retinaculum.

3. No, there is no communication with the ankle joint.

4. Shallow or convex fibular groove or laxity of the superior peroneal retinaculum.

Reference

Khoury NJ, El-Khoury GY, Saltzman CL, Kathol MH: Peroneus longus and brevis tendon tears: MR imaging evaluation. Radiology 200:833–841, 1996.

Comments

The majority of peroneal tendon tears are partial and oriented in the long axis of the tendon, splitting the tendon into two or more bundles. Note that in this patient portions of the peroneus brevis tendon straddle the peroneus longus tendon. Unsuspected tears can be a source of chronic pain and instability and may require surgical repair. Tears of the peroneus brevis tendon can be caused by numerous mechanisms and have a high prevalence among young, athletic people as well as among elderly people. When related to trauma, the mechanism of injury is forceful dorsiflexion with inversion of the foot. Magnetic resonance imaging is ideal for evaluating the peroneal tendons because it allows multiplanar assessment of these tendons but also because it is highly sensitive to inflammatory changes in and about the tendon. The hallmark of acute tears of the peroneal tendons on magnetic resonance images is increased signal intensity within the substance of the tendon on T1W and T2W images, appearing as a linear area of altered signal. The tendon may also be thickened focally in a fusiform fashion depending on the length of the tear and the chronicity of the injury. In chronic tears, the changes in signal intensity may be less intense on T2W images, although a thickened morphology usually persists and may be even more exaggerated than in the acute phase of the tear, owing to the development of fibrosis.

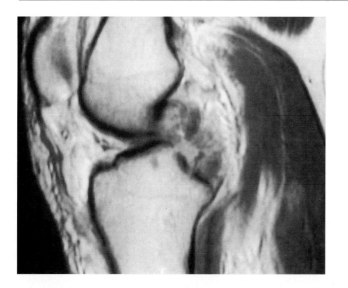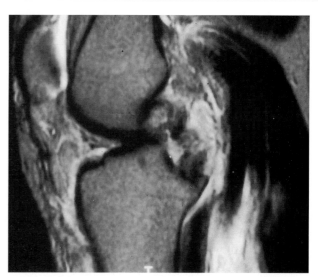

1. What are the likely mechanisms of injury?

2. What two structures may be found adjacent to this ligament?

3. Where do ruptures of this ligament commonly occur?

4. What other injuries are usually associated with this injury?

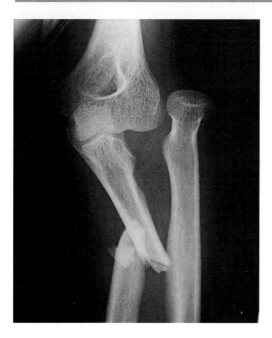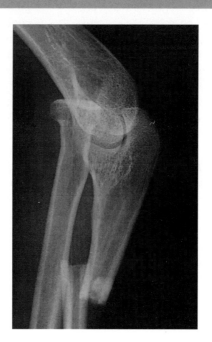

1. Name this injury. Is it common?

2. What are some potential complications of this fracture-dislocation injury?

3. What is a variation of this lesion that is more common in children?

4. What is Galeazzi's lesion?

Posterior Cruciate Ligament Tear

1. Hyperextension, direct impaction on the anterior tibia with knee flexion, knee dislocations, and rotational injuries.

2. The meniscofemoral ligaments of Humphrey (anterior) and Wrisberg (posterior).

3. Fifty to seventy-five percent midsubstance, 30% to 35% femur avulsion, 20% to 30% tibia avulsion.

4. Meniscal tears and injuries to the anterior cruciate or collateral ligaments.

Reference

Grover JS, Bassett LW, Gross ML, et al: Posterior cruciate ligament: MR imaging. Radiology 174:527-530, 1990.

Comments

The posterior cruciate ligament (PCL) is the primary stabilizer of the knee joint against posterior translation of the tibia or excessive external rotation of the femur. It attaches proximally to the lateral aspect of the medial femoral condyle and courses in a posterior direction to attach distally in the posterior tibia near its cortex. It is composed of two important bands; the anterolateral band that tightens when the knee flexes and the posteromedial band that tightens when the knee extends. On magnetic resonance imaging, the appearance of the PCL is a tubular arc of uniform low signal intensity with a cross-sectional diameter measuring 1 cm. Aside from the meniscofemoral ligaments and the anterior cruciate ligament, only fat surrounds the cruciate sheath. When examining magnetic resonance images of the PCL, one must scrutinize both the morphology and the signal intensity of this ligament. Acute tears disrupt the morphology, resulting in surface irregularities, gaps with frayed ends, focal thickening or attenuation, or an osseous avulsion. Acutely, the change in morphology is associated with interstitial edema and hemorrhage, seen as areas of high signal intensity on T2W images, and occasionally with marrow edema if the bone attachment has been avulsed. There may also be injuries to the secondary posterolateral restraining structures of the knee, which include the posterolateral capsule and the popliteus tendon. Chronic tears are more difficult to identify because low signal intensity fibrous tissue may fill in the ligament defect. In these situations, any change in morphology should be closely evaluated.

Monteggia's Lesion

1. Monteggia's lesion (type 3). No, it constitutes less than 1% of elbow injuries.

2. Diminished range of motion from heterotopic ossification, median and ulnar nerve injury, and injury to the brachial artery.

3. Anterior dislocation of the radial head without a fracture of the ulna or with an epiphyseal fracture of a dislocated radial head.

4. Fracture of the distal radius with dislocation of the distal radioulnar joint.

Reference

Bado JL: The Monteggia lesion. Clin Orthop 50:71-86, 1967.

Comments

Monteggia's lesion is a complex injury that is composed of a fracture of the ulnar shaft associated with a dislocation of the radial head. Bado classified this injury complex into four types. A type 1 Monteggia's lesion, the most common type (it accounts for 60% of fracture-dislocations in this group), is characterized by anterior angulation of the ulnar fracture and an anterior dislocation of the radial head. Posterior angulation of the ulnar fracture and posterior dislocation of the radial head characterize a type 2 Monteggia's lesion (10% to 15%). A type 3 Monteggia's lesion (6% to 20%) is characterized by a fracture of the proximal ulna occurring distal to the coronoid process of the ulna and by a lateral dislocation of the radial head. The least common type is a type 4 Monteggia's fracture (5%), which is characterized by a fracture of the proximal ends of both the radius and the ulna and an anterior dislocation of the radial head. The mechanism of injury and the direction of the impaction force dictate the type of fracture seen. The most common complication of Monteggia's fracture-dislocation is recurrent dislocation of the radial head.

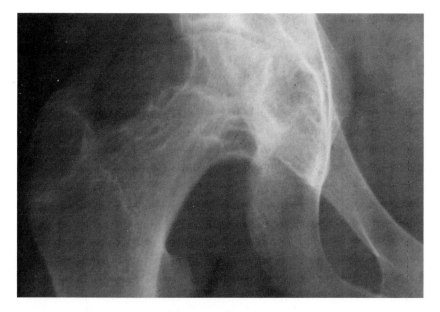

1. What is the dominant finding in this case?
2. What is the differential diagnosis?
3. Is hypertrophic osteophyte formation a typical feature of pigmented villonodular synovitis (PVNS)?
4. On magnetic resonance imaging, what would you see in patients with PVNS?

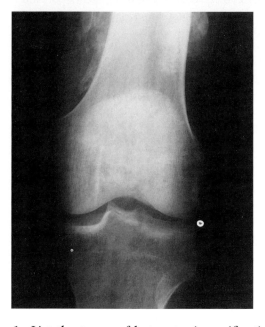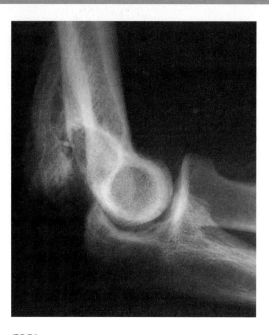

1. List the types of heterotopic ossification (HO).
2. What are the necessary factors needed to form new bone?
3. Does the formation of HO cause symptoms?
4. When does HO begin? When can we detect it?

Pigmented Villonodular Synovitis

1. Multiple juxta-articular, cystlike erosions in the non–weight-bearing region of the femoral head and neck and the acetabulum.

2. PVNS, osteochondromatosis, and any other intra-articular process that can cause osseous erosion.

3. No.

4. Masses of low signal intensity on T1W and variable signal intensity on T2W images, hemosiderin deposition, joint effusion, and well-defined erosions.

References

Cotton A, Flipo RM, Chastanet P, et al: Pigmented villo-nodular synovitis of the hip: Review of radiographic features in 58 patients. Skeletal Radiol 24:1–6, 1995.

Dorwart RH, Genant HK, Johnston WH, Morris JM: Pigmented villonodular synovitis of synovial joints: Clinical, pathologic, and radiologic features. AJR Am J Roentgenol 143:877–885, 1984.

Comments

This patient has PVNS. Villonodular synovitis is a proliferative disorder affecting the synovium of joints, bursae, and tendons. Patients with this condition are usually young adults between the ages of 20 and 40 years. Patients present with chronic pain, diminished range of motion, and intermittent joint locking. The pathogenesis is unknown, although theories support both neoplastic and inflammatory processes. PVNS is the diffuse form of villonodular synovitis and is so named because the extensive deposition of hemosiderin gives the lesion a brownish appearance on gross pathologic inspection. A hemorrhagic effusion is a common finding; it appears denser than other effusions radiographically. The hallmark of this process is numerous bony erosions, which are variable in size, surrounded by sclerotic rims, and localized to a juxta-articular distribution. Calcifications are not typical. Periarticular osteopenia is indicative of the hypervascular nature of this process. Loss of joint space may be concentric or localized, but this is not a dominant feature of the disease; a lack of an osteophytic response is a notable finding.

The differential diagnosis includes synovial osteo-chondromatosis; however, intra-articular bodies and lack of joint effusion are dominant features of this condition. Intra-articular masses such as lipoma arborescens and synovial hemangiomas are rare. Other intra-articular processes, such as rheumatoid arthritis, osteoarthritis, and crystal deposition arthropathies, have specific features that permit differentiation.

Heterotopic Ossification

1. There are three forms: traumatic, neurogenic, and myositis ossificans progressiva.

2. Three factors are required: osteogenic precursor cell, inducing agent or agents, and environment that permits formation of new bone.

3. Yes, pain and diminished range of motion. Swelling, fever, erythema, and a palpable mass may mimic infection or deep venous thrombosis.

4. Approximately 2 weeks after the primary insult. Bone scintigraphy becomes positive at 3 weeks, and radiographs show early signs of ossification after about 4 to 6 weeks when osteoid mineralization occurs.

References

Feldman F: Soft tissue mineralization: Roentgen analysis. Curr Probl Diagn Radiol 15:161–240, 1986.

Moed BR, Smith ST: Three-view radiographic assessment of heterotopic ossification after acetabular fracture surgery. J Orthop Trauma 10:93–98, 1996.

Comments

HO is a well-recognized condition characterized by the formation of mature, lamellar bone in the soft tissues. There are three forms of HO. Traumatic HO occurs after fractures and dislocations or after procedures such as total hip replacements and internal fixation of fractures. Neurogenic HO occurs after traumatic brain injuries, spinal cord trauma, strokes, or infections and tumors that affect the central nervous system. Myositis ossificans progressiva is a rare hereditary disease (autosomal dominant) characterized by the progressive deposition of heterotopic bone throughout the skeleton. This patient had a traumatic brain injury sustained during a motor vehicle accident. In neurogenic HO, ossification appears about 2 to 6 months after the initial insult. Common areas affected are the hips, shoulders, knees, and elbows, and more than one site may be involved. Initially, the HO appears as an ill-defined radiodense area, lacking in trabeculation. As it enlarges, the cortex and trabeculation become apparent. Bridging HO may cause complete ankylosis of a joint. Treatment has two different goals. The first is prophylaxis, and it may involve administration of nonsteroidal anti-inflammatory drugs or radiation therapy. The second is restoring motion of the involved joint after the HO has completely matured (based on the absence of activity on bone scintigraphy).

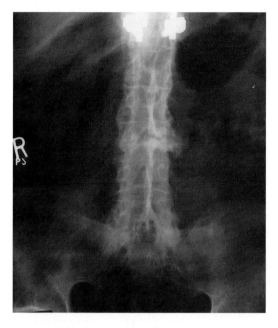

1. What is the diagnosis?
2. How do these patients present?
3. Clinically, what are important diagnostic considerations?
4. What would you see on magnetic resonance imaging? Would you be able to exclude infection?

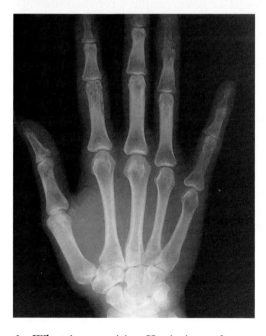 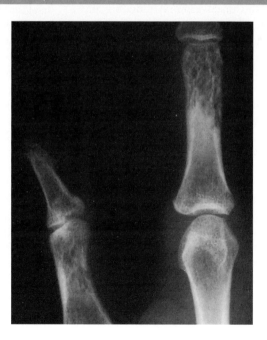

1. What is a positive Kveim's test?
2. Would you expect any abnormal laboratory serum levels in this patient?
3. How frequently are the joints involved in this condition? Characterize the different arthropathies.
4. What is the typical appearance of skull lesions? Which skull table is involved?

Pseudoarthrosis in Ankylosing Spondylitis

1. Ankylosing spondylitis (AS) with pseudoarthrosis of the lumbar spine.

2. New-onset back pain, often after minor trauma.

3. Acute transdiscal fracture and infectious diskitis.

4. Low signal intensity on T1W images and heterogeneous signal intensity on T2W images from granulation tissue (hyperintense) and fibrous tissue (hypointense) as well as paraspinal soft-tissue swelling. It is difficult to exclude infection without a biopsy, but in this patient the adjacent end plates above and below the pseudoarthrosis appear normal, excluding diskitis.

Reference

Vitellas KM, Yu JS, Oehler M: Ankylosing spondylitis complicated by pseudoarthrosis and secondary spinal stenosis. Emergency Radiol 5:113-115, 1998.

Comments

This patient has AS. The sacroiliac joints are ankylosed, as are the disk spaces, facet joints, and interspinous ligaments. The increased rigidity of the spine renders patients with long-standing AS susceptible to minor trauma, leading to the development of a pseudoarthrosis. The most common etiology of a pseudoarthrosis is a fracture through the discovertebral junction and apophyseal articulation. Abnormal motion evolves into a fibrous nonunion. Penetration and proliferation of fibrovascular granulation tissue from the intervertebral disk into the vertebra cause destruction of the end plates. The thoracolumbar junction is the most common site of a pseudoarthrosis because it is the area of the spine that sustains the greatest amount of stress.

A pseudoarthrosis is an important complication of AS that results in severe, disabling back pain; deformity; and neurologic deficit. It should be considered when patients develop back pain, particularly after trauma, because in the course of the disease back pain generally diminishes as the spine becomes ankylosed. Spinal cord impingement caused by hypertrophic osseous and ligamentous changes, retropulsed bone fragments, or epidural inflammation is a serious condition. Computed tomography and magnetic resonance imaging can identify complications such as spinal stenosis and ligamentous disruption. The differential diagnosis includes an acute transdiscal fracture and infectious diskitis. An acute transdiscal fracture, occurring most commonly at the lower cervical spine, is not associated with end plate erosions and is often accompanied by an epidural hematoma. Infectious diskitis may be more difficult to differentiate (it may require a biopsy), but marrow edema is suggestive.

Sarcoidosis

1. Intradermal injection with a suspension of sarcoidosis tissue elicits a nodule of noncaseating granulomas.

2. Calcium and alkaline phosphatase levels are frequently elevated.

3. About 10% to 35% of patients. Acute synovial inflammatory polyarthritis (small and medium joints) of short duration (4 to 6 weeks) and chronic polyarthritis (lasting months to years) producing irreversible joint destruction and disability.

4. Single or multiple small, lytic lesions with no surrounding rim of sclerosis. Lesions affect both inner and outer tables.

References

Hall FM, Shmerling RH, Aronson M, Faix JD: Case report 705. Osteosclerotic sarcoidosis. Skeletal Radiol 21:182-185, 1992.

Smith K, Fort JG: Phalangeal osseous sarcoidosis. Arthritis Rheum 41:176-179, 1998.

Comments

Sarcoidosis is a systemic granulomatous condition of unknown etiology. This disorder affects multiple organ systems, and the skin, eyes, lungs, lymph nodes, liver, gastrointestinal tract, brain, nerves, and bones are the usual target sites. In young people, a common presentation of sarcoidosis is hilar and paratracheal adenopathy, erythema nodosum, and uveitis. Three to ten percent of patients affected have osseous manifestations during the course of the disease, and these tend to occur concurrently with cutaneous disease. The osseous lesions of sarcoidosis are typically painless. The tubular bones of the hands and feet are common locations. Sarcoidosis of bone has three radiographic forms. The diffuse form is characterized by generalized osteopenia associated with thinning and striations of the cortex (related to granulomatous destruction and replacement of the trabeculation in the spongiosa), resulting in a lacy medullary appearance. The circumscribed form is characterized by punched-out cystic lesions measuring up to 5 mm in diameter. When these cystic lesions coalesce, they can evolve into a mutilating form, characterized by rapid bone destruction and cortical disruption. Less commonly, areas of osteosclerosis may occur in the tubular bones of the hands and feet (acro-osteosclerosis). Rarely, this process can become widespread in the skeleton, mimicking blastic metastasis.

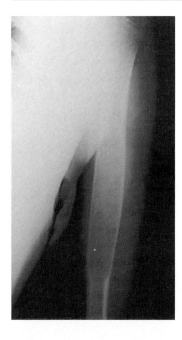
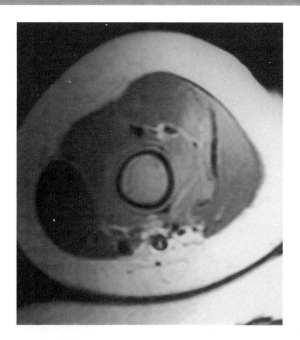
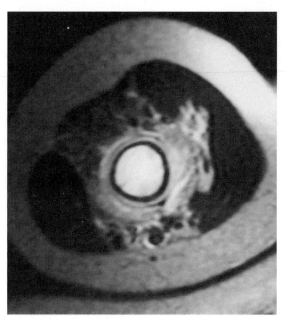
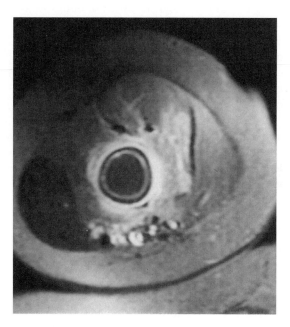

1. What entities did you consider based on the radiographic findings?

2. Can Ewing's sarcoma arise in the epiphysis?

3. What are the two least common radiographic presentations of Ewing's sarcoma?

4. What radiographic findings of Ewing's sarcoma can mimic those of an osteosarcoma?

Ewing's Sarcoma

1. Fibrous dysplasia, eosinophilic granuloma, Ewing's sarcoma, neuroblastoma metastasis, and low-grade intraosseous osteosarcoma.

2. Ten percent of Ewing's sarcomas extend to the epiphysis, but pure epiphyseal involvement is rare.

3. "Normal" radiographs from diffuse involvement (rare) and a well-marginated lesion (less than 4%).

4. Marked reactive (sclerotic) bone in 15% of cases.

References

Enneking WF: Staging of musculoskeletal neoplasms. Skeletal Radiol 13:183–194, 1985.

Ma LD, Frassica FJ, Scott WW, et al: Differentiation of benign and malignant musculoskeletal tumors: Potential pitfalls with MR imaging. Radiographics 15:349–366, 1995.

Comments

Ewing's sarcoma is a common malignant tumor of bone. It accounts for about 10% of all primary bone tumors. Nearly 95% of patients are between the ages of 4 and 25 years at presentation, with a peak age between 10 and 15 years. Males are twice as likely to be affected. Pain is the presenting symptom in half of patients; it is initially characterized as intermittent but increases in severity over time. Frequently, patients may present with nonspecific symptoms, such as fever, increased erythrocyte sedimentation rate, and leukocytosis, that suggest an infection, or the patient may present with weight loss and anemia. There may be a significant delay in rendering a diagnosis owing to the indolent nature of this tumor early in the disease. As a result, by the time the tumor is discovered, 15% to 30% of patients have evidence of metastases. The pelvis and long bones are involved in 75% of cases, but the spine (usually the sacrum) may be involved in 6% of patients.

The radiographic findings demonstrated by this patient are uncommon; they represent one of the least common presentations of this tumor, a well-marginated lesion. More typical findings of Ewing's sarcoma are poor margination, permeative or moth-eaten osteolysis, cortical erosion, exuberant periostitis, and soft-tissue mass. Osteosclerosis (mimicking osteosarcoma) and sequestration (mimicking osteomyelitis) can be confusing observations. The magnetic resonance imaging findings are typical. Ewing's sarcomas are frequently found to be more extensive than expected because radiographs usually underestimate the tumor size.

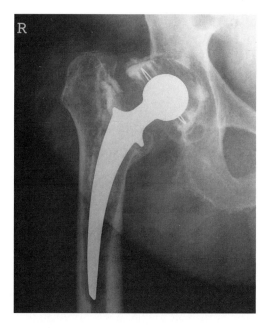
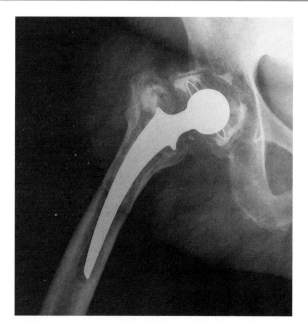

1. What is the primary factor that stimulates new bone formation around a total joint prosthesis?

2. List some factors that can lead to bone resorption.

3. What is the hypothesized effect of cytokines on this condition?

4. What radiographic findings are most helpful in identifying an infected prosthesis?

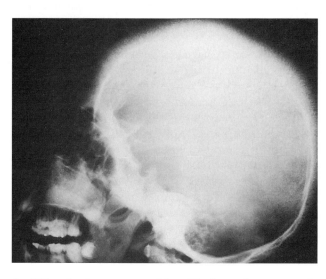
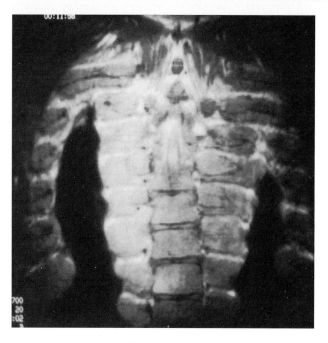

1. What is the process identified on the magnetic resonance image, and what diseases would you consider?

2. How may other organs may be affected in this disease?

3. Where does the "hair-on-end" appearance begin in the skull, and what does it represent?

4. If the patient has right upper quadrant abdominal pain, what should be done?

Particle-Related Inflammatory Disease

1. Mechanical load.

2. Infection, particle disease, insufficient mechanical load, and implant motion.

3. It probably acts directly on osteoclasts or on its precursors.

4. Ill-defined periprosthetic resorption, acute periosteal reaction, and multiple sites of subacute periosteal reaction.

Reference

Bauer TW, Schils J: The pathology of total joint arthroplasty. II. Mechanisms of implant failure. Skeletal Radiol 28:483–497, 1999.

Comments

Periprosthetic lucency around hip arthroplasties is an important radiologic observation. It is the most common radiographic sign of loosening, and, in this situation, a zone of lucency more than 2 mm thick outlines the prosthesis. However, progressive widening of this lucency and cement fractures are strong indicators of loosening. There are other causes of radiolucency about the components of a hip replacement. One of these causes is particle-related inflammatory disease (aggressive granulomatosis), a condition characterized by rapid and progressive resorption of bone. It can be unifocal or multifocal.

The condition occurs when small metal, methylmethacrylate, or polyethylene fragments induce a foreign-body reaction. Macrophages become activated after exposure to a foreign material. The release of cytokines, such as tumor necrosis factor, further contributes to bone loss around the prosthetic device, ultimately causing its failure through loosening and the development of stress fractures. Foreign-body–type giant cells also participate in this condition, as do osteoclasts. The differential diagnosis includes infection. In this situation, aspiration of the hip joint is required for diagnosis.

Extramedullary Hematopoiesis (Thalassemia Major)

1. Extramedullary hematopoiesis. Thalassemia, sickle cell disease, hereditary spherocytosis, and elliptocytosis.

2. Hepatosplenomegaly, cardiomegaly, skeletal dwarfism, and delayed sex characteristics.

3. Frontal bones. Thinning and external displacement of the outer table.

4. Ultrasound to look for gallstones.

Reference

Tsitouridis J, Stamos S, Hassapopoulou E, et al: Extramedullary paraspinal hematopoiesis in thalassemia: CT and MRI evaluation. Eur J Radiol 30:33–38, 1999.

Comments

Extramedullary hematopoiesis commonly occurs in thalassemia and may present as a paraspinal soft-tissue mass. It represents a compensatory mechanism that occurs when the blood-forming organs cannot supply an adequate volume of red blood cells required by the body. Patients with polycythemia, myelofibrosis, leukemia, Hodgkin's disease, and other marrow-replacement processes occasionally demonstrate a need for extramedullary hematopoiesis. The radiographic appearance of intrathoracic extramedullary hematopoiesis is that of a paraspinal mass in the posterior mediastinum at the level of the middle to lower thorax. The process may be either unilateral or bilateral. These masses generally appear rounded or lobulated and do not contain calcifications. Neurologic symptoms from spinal cord involvement are rare.

The differential diagnosis includes a number of entities that may occur in the posterior mediastinum. Of note, neural tumors may contain some calcification but, more importantly, frequently demonstrate erosive or destructive changes in the adjacent bone. A tuberculous abscess may be associated with a compression (gibbus) deformity of a vertebral body. A teratoma often contains adipose tissue and calcifications but is unlikely to be a bilateral process. The key to the diagnosis is the skull radiograph. Although a diffuse "hair-on-end" appearance occurs in a number of diseases, thalassemia is the only condition that also causes maxillary hypertrophy with forward displacement of the incisors, producing a characteristic "rodent facies" appearance.

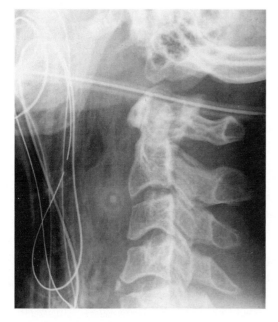

1. How common is this injury, and what is its usual outcome?
2. What is the proposed mechanism of injury?
3. How is the diagnosis confirmed on the radiograph?
4. Is this injury more common in children or in adults, and why?

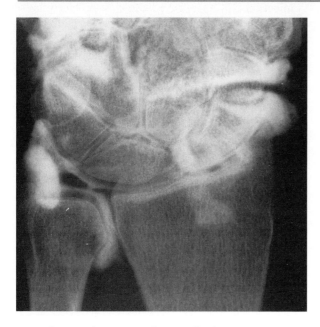

1. What is this procedure called? How many injections are required in a normal study?
2. What is the diagnosis?
3. How would you diagnose a triangular fibrocartilage (TFC) detachment? What do you look for?
4. What is the relationship between degenerative perforations and age?

Occipitocervical Dissociation

1. Rare, nearly universally lethal (brainstem injury).

2. Extreme hyperextension of the neck with a second distractive force acting on the head.

3. By a Powers ratio greater than 1.

4. More common in children because their condyles are smaller and because the articular relationship of the condyles to the lateral masses of C1 is more horizontal.

Reference

Woodring JH, Selke AC, Duff DE: Traumatic atlanto-occipital dislocation with survival. AJR Am J Roentgenol 137:21–24, 1991.

Comments

The injury sustained by this patient is rare, and few patients survive this type of dislocation. It is caused either by significant distractive forces applied to the head when the neck is hyperextended or by a shearing injury to the face or to the occipital region of the skull. Both mechanisms can cause rupture of the tectorial membrane and alar ligaments of the occipitoatlantoaxial joints and usually require a high-velocity force, such as those sustained during a motor vehicle accident. The diagnosis is relatively straightforward and is based on observations obtained from the lateral radiograph of the cervical spine. The Powers ratio defines a normal relationship between the base of the skull and the atlas. In this ratio, the length of a line drawn from the basion to the spinolaminar line of C1 divided by the length of a line drawn from the opisthion to the posterior margin of the anterior arch of C1 is determined. If the ratio is less than 1, no dislocation exists. However, if the ratio exceeds 1, then a dislocation is present. The treatment of choice if a patient survives this injury is surgical stabilization by occipito-C2 arthrodesis followed by ha-lothoracic immobilization for at least 12 weeks.

Triangular Fibrocartilage Tear

1. Three-phase wrist arthrogram. Three (midcarpal compartment, radiocarpal joint, and distal radioulnar joint [DRUJ]).

2. TFC tear.

3. Direct injection of the DRUJ. Look for extravasation of contrast into the ulnar soft tissues.

4. Linear—they increase linearly with each decade after the second decade of life.

Reference

Levingsohn EM: Imaging of the wrist. Radiol Clin North Am 28:905–921, 1990.

Comments

The radiocarpal joint, midcarpal compartment, and DRUJ do not normally communicate with one another. Most experts agree that using a three-phase arthrogram instead of a one-injection study increases the likelihood of demonstrating ligamentous or TFC perforations, with one study indicating that up to 30% more abnormalities are discovered. Perforation of the TFC is a common injury and accounts for about 25% of patients with ulnar-sided wrist pain, whereas a TFC detachment accounts for 15% of cases. Another 10% to 15% of patients present with a proximal surface defect identified by a DRUJ injection. TFC tears have been classified into three types. Type 1 tears (40%) involve the radial half of the disk. Type 2 tears are the most common type (50%) and involve the central portion of the disk. They have a high association with chondromalacia of the lunate. Type 3 tears (10%) involve the ulnar half of the disk. Nearly one third of people with painful wrists have been shown to have communications between the midcarpal and radiocarpal compartments, indicating an abnormality of one or both proximal intercarpal ligaments.

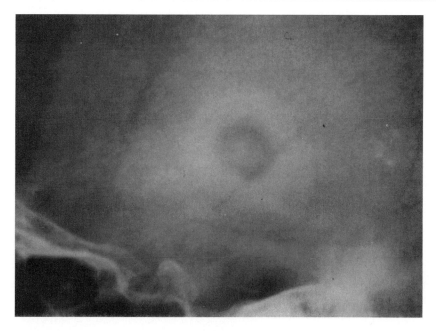

1. What is your differential diagnosis?
2. Would you consider cystic tuberculosis in this patient?
3. What can cause this appearance in a carpal or tarsal bone?
4. When is a lytic metastasis likely to become sclerotic?

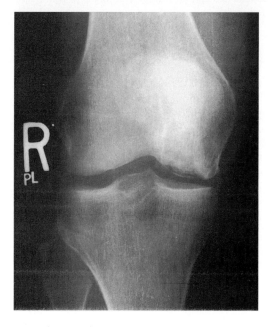
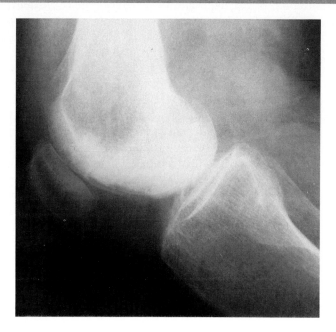

1. What is the diagnosis? What else did you consider?
2. What are associated risk factors for this condition?
3. When do subchondral fractures become apparent in the majority of cases?
4. In the acute phase of the disease, what imaging modality would you choose to make the diagnosis, magnetic resonance imaging (MRI) or bone scan?

Button Sequestrum

1. Eosinophilic granuloma, pyogenic osteomyelitis, radiation necrosis, Paget's disease, and osseous metastasis.

2. Only at the end of the list. Cystic tuberculosis can produce a round lesion in the skull with a rim of sclerosis, but it usually does not contain a central radiodense focus.

3. Osteoid osteoma.

4. After the patient has undergone chemotherapy or radiation therapy.

References

Rosen IW, Nadel HI: Button sequestrum of the skull. Radiology 92:969-971, 1969.

Satin R, Usher MS, Goldenberg M: More causes of button sequestrum. J Can Assoc Radiol 27:288-289, 1976.

Comments

A button sequestrum is defined as a radiodense focus within a lytic cranial lesion, with or without surrounding sclerosis. The margins of the lesion may be sharply demarcated or slightly ill defined. It is common in patients with eosinophilic granuloma, where extension into the dura or the brain can occur. Nonuniform growth of the lesion can lead to beveled margins and unequal destruction of the inner and outer tables. Osteomyelitis can result in this radiographic appearance. The central sequestrum is frequently sharply marginated, and the sclerosis is related to an interrupted blood supply that prevents its participation in the hyperemic osteopenia of the adjacent bone. Radiation therapy may cause focal osteonecrosis, particularly if the dose exceeds 3600 rads. Paget's disease of the skull is referred to as osteoporosis circumscripta, reflecting the osteolytic form of the disease, and this may surround a radiodense focus of bone. Metastasis may produce this type of lesion de novo or after treatment. Sclerosis of a lytic metastasis after radiation therapy or chemotherapy tends to begin at the periphery of the lesion. Disseminated cystic tuberculosis, multiple myeloma, sarcoidosis, epidermoid cysts, cystic angiomatosis, and prominent venous lakes may produce lytic lesions in the skull with or without surrounding sclerosis, but these conditions typically lack a central sclerotic focus.

Spontaneous Osteonecrosis of the Knee

1. Spontaneous osteonecrosis of the knee. Osteochondritis dissecans, posttraumatic osteochondral defect, and neuroarthropathy.

2. Obesity, trauma, corticosteroid administration, and meniscal tears.

3. Six to 9 months from the onset of symptoms.

4. MRI is preferred over bone scintigraphy owing to its superior spatial resolution.

References

Bjorkengren AG, Al-Rowaih A, Lindstrand A, et al: Spontaneous osteonecrosis of the knee: Value of MR imaging in determining prognosis. AJR Am J Roentgenol 154:331-336, 1990.

Valenti N, Jr, Leyes M, Schweitzer D: Spontaneous osteonecrosis of the knee. Treatment and evolution. Knee Surg Sports Traumatol Arthrosc 6:12-15, 1998.

Comments

Spontaneous osteonecrosis of the knee is a distinct clinical entity that occurs predominantly over the load-bearing surface of the medial femoral condyle. Most patients are elderly, the majority presenting at older than 50 years, and this condition has its highest incidence in the sixth and seventh decades of life. The hallmark of this disease is a sudden onset of pain, and an association with the development of a meniscal tear has been suggested. In some patients, the disease evolves quickly, resulting in collapse of the articular surface and development of secondary osteoarthritis. Initial radiographs obtained during the acute phase of the disease are often normal. However, soon after the acute phase, flattening of the weight-bearing surface of the medial femoral condyle develops, and a narrow zone of increased density reflecting trabecular compression surrounds the devitalized area. Over time, a radiolucent crescent in the subchondral bone becomes evident (a clue that should always be sought after). As the lesion progresses, joint space narrowing, subchondral eburnation, and development of periostitis and osteophytosis may eventually obscure some or all of the features of osteonecrosis.

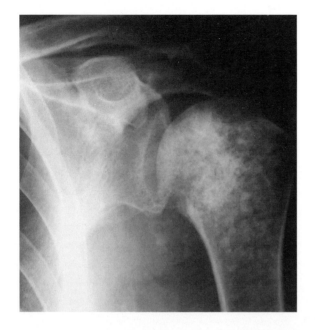
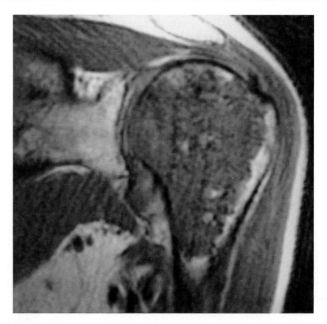

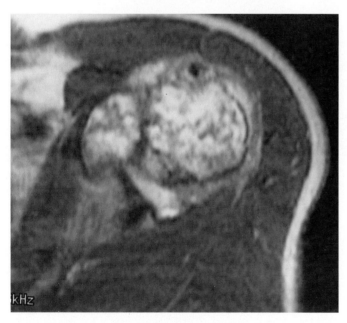

1. What is the differential diagnosis?

2. What key observation enabled you to narrow your differential diagnosis on the radiograph?

3. How would you describe chondroid calcifications? Do this patient's calcifications fit the description?

4. List the aggressive features of this patient's neoplasm.

Chondrosarcoma

1. Chondrosarcoma, enchondroma, lymphoma, and metastasis.

2. Cortical break in the medial aspect of the humeral neck and calcifications in the axillary pouch that represented tumor extension on magnetic resonance imaging (MRI).

3. Amorphous, punctate, dense, or irregular. Yes.

4. Large (5 cm); endosteal scalloping; cortical breakthrough; soft-tissue mass; and wide zone of transition. On MRI, heterogeneously bright signal intensity on T2W images.

Reference

Mandell GA, Harcke HT, Kumar SJ: Chondroid lesions of the extremities. Top Magn Reson Imaging 4:56–65, 1991.

Comments

Chondrosarcoma is a malignant tumor of cartilaginous origin. It may be a primary lesion or may develop from a pre-existing cartilage-containing lesion such as an osteochondroma or enchondroma. These tumors may be categorized according to location (central, peripheral, juxtacortical), degree of cellular differentiation (low grade, medium grade, high grade), or unusual histologic features (mesenchymal, clear cell). Central chondrosarcomas are more common than are the peripheral type, and primary tumors are more common than are secondary lesions. Chondrosarcomas may occur at any age, but 50% of tumors affect people who are older than 40 years. Males and females are nearly equally affected. A dull ache or pain is the most common presenting complaint, and it may be present for 1 to 2 years before the tumor is discovered. The long tubular bones (50% of cases) and the innominate bones of the pelvis, ribs, vertebra, sternum, and scapula are common sites of involvement. The radiographic manifestation is strongly influenced by the location of the tumor. Central chondrosarcomas often present as an expansile, lytic, well-marginated mass with endosteal thinning or thickening. When the tumor growth exceeds the rate of osseous repair, the lesion appears poorly marginated. Cortical destruction and invasion of the soft tissues produce a large soft-tissue mass with calcifications (note that in this patient the mass has invaded the joint space on the T2W axial image).

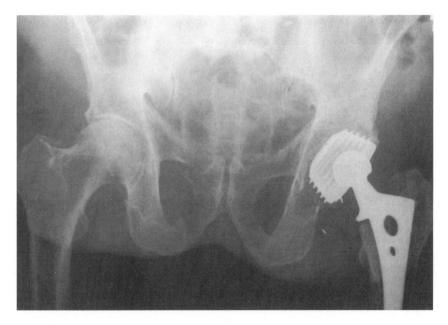

1. What do you see?
2. Who is at risk for developing this condition?
3. List some potential complications of this fracture.
4. Clinically, what is the most important diagnostic consideration that must be excluded?

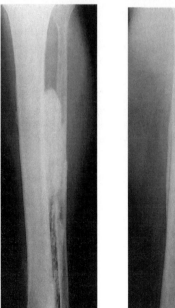
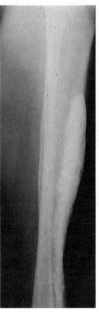
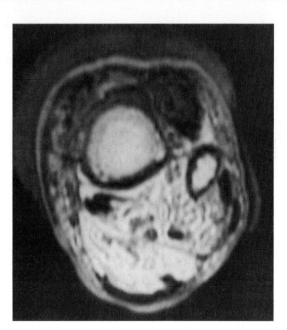

1. List the differential considerations.
2. How does one arrive at a diagnosis of acute compartment syndrome? What is required for this syndrome to occur?
3. What is chronic or recurrent compartment syndrome?
4. When does neuromuscular damage occur in acute compartment syndrome?

C A S E 1 5 0

Stress Fracture Complicating Total Hip Arthroplasty

1. Stress fracture of the pubic ramus.

2. Long-distance runners (fatigue fracture) and patients with total hip arthroplasty, femur fracture reduction, osteoporosis, rheumatoid arthritis, or osteoarthritis (insufficiency fracture).

3. Osteolysis (mimics a malignancy), delayed union, development of other fractures in the pelvis.

4. Infection involving the arthroplasty.

Reference

Torisu T, Izumi H, Fujikawa Y, Masumi S: Bipolar hip arthroplasty without acetabular bone-grafting for dysplastic osteoarthritis. Results after 6-9 years. J Arthroplasty 10:15-27, 1995.

Comments

Stress fractures involving the pubic bone are infrequent but are relatively common in patients who have had previous hip surgery such as hip arthroplasty or fracture reduction of the proximal femur. Classically, patients present with new-onset, moderate to severe hip or groin pain that is aggravated by motion. On physical examination, a patient may walk with a limp and have local tenderness that is difficult to characterize and that is often dismissed as a muscle strain. Development of stress fractures of the pubic bone may be precipitated by altered gait, which may be further exacerbated by either disuse or senile osteoporosis. Increased activity after surgery can also exert additional forces after a period of immobilization. Stress fracture in patients who have had a hip arthroplasty usually affects only one side of the pelvis, and these fractures heal without difficulty. The most common site is the inferior pubic ramus, although fracture may also occur in the superior pubic ramus, the superior acetabular region of the ilium, and either side of the sacrum. Diagnosis is not difficult with sequential radiographs because an obvious deformity with the formation of callus develops at the fracture site. The fracture, however, can be detected earlier either with bone scintigraphy or magnetic resonance imaging. Both techniques are more sensitive to stress fractures than conventional radiography is.

C A S E 1 5 1

Anterior Compartment Syndrome

1. Anterior compartment syndrome, calcific myonecrosis, and myositis ossificans.

2. The symptoms are intense pain, with loss of sensation and motor function, and increased intramuscular pressure exceeding 50 mm Hg. An inelastic limiting envelope (fascia) and increased tissue pressure within the compartment (edema, hemorrhage, or both) are required.

3. Condition in which exercise elevates the intramuscular pressure in the anterior compartment of the lower extremity enough to cause transient ischemia but not enough to cause myonecrosis.

4. If the obstruction is relieved within 4 hours, the injury is reversible. If it is not restored within 12 hours, it is almost always permanent. Between 4 and 12 hours, results are variable.

Reference

Yu JS: MR imaging of soft tissue trauma. Emerg Radiol 3:181-194, 1996.

Comments

Compartment syndrome is characterized by a sudden increase in the intramuscular pressure of a fascial compartment in the upper or lower extremity. If left untreated, the condition can progress to myonecrosis because of the interference in blood flow to the muscles. A variety of situations can cause massive muscle swelling in a compartment, such as trauma, bleeding disorders, prolonged tourniquet application, and major vascular injury. The sequelae to acute compartment syndrome include fibrosis and contracture of the extremity and permanent neurologic deficit. Magnetic resonance imaging is well suited for detecting the extent of rhabdomyolysis in patients with clinical evidence of acute compartment syndrome, but obtaining the examination should not delay treatment because the interval of time for decompression is critical. Necrotic muscle demonstrates lengthening of the T2 relaxation time, which allows clear demarcation of viable muscle from regions that require débridement on T2W images. When the condition is left untreated or becomes chronic, sheetlike collections of calcification develop at the site of tissue injury (as in this case).

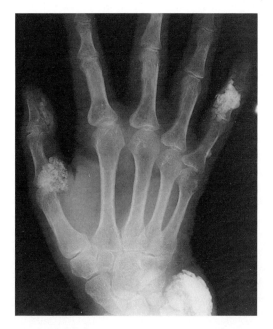 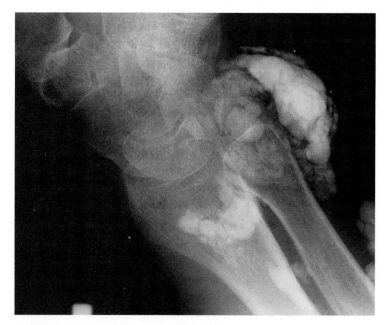

1. What are the likely considerations if you note the numerous soft-tissue masses?
2. Can intra-articular corticosteroid injections produce soft-tissue calcifications?
3. What is milk-alkali syndrome?
4. How much vitamin D needs to be ingested to elicit the clinical manifestations of acute hypervitaminosis D? What are some symptoms?

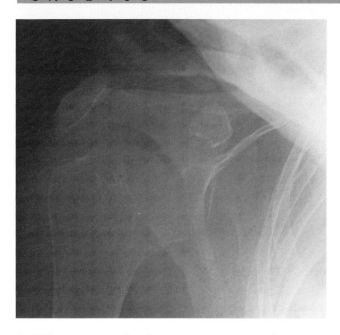 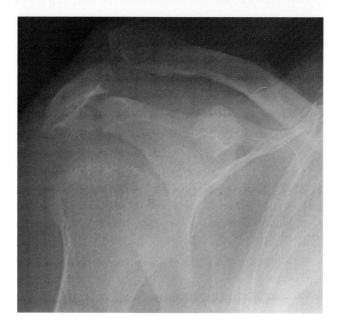

1. Why are scapular fractures uncommon?
2. How does scapulothoracic dissociation appear radiographically?
3. The acromion process usually develops from how many ossification centers?
4. What other injuries should you look for when you identify a displaced acromion process fracture? What nerve is at risk?

Secondary Tumoral Calcinosis

1. Scleroderma, hyperparathyroidism, renal osteodystrophy, hypervitaminosis D, milk-alkali syndrome, dermatomyositis, polymyositis, and sarcoidosis.

2. Yes.

3. Hypercalcemia without hypercalciuria or hypophosphatemia caused by excessive intake of milk and alkali for treatment of chronic peptic ulcer disease.

4. Four to 18 million units per day for about a week. Vomiting, cramps, fever, dehydration, bone pain, thirst, anorexia, and polyuria.

Reference

Steinbach LS, Johnston JO, Tepper EF, et al: Tumoral calcinosis: Radiologic-pathologic correlation. Skeletal Radiol 24:573–578, 1995.

Comments

The main observation in this case is the presence of tumorous periarticular soft-tissue calcifications, resembling soft-tissue masses. When evaluating these masses, it is useful to consider overlap syndromes such as scleroderma and dermatomyositis or systemic lupus erythematosus. Amorphous calcifications in patients with scleroderma are common, especially in the digits, occurring in 10% to 30% of cases. Hypervitaminosis D and milk-alkali syndrome are not common but remain important considerations, emphasizing the importance of a complete medical history. In calcium pyrophosphate crystal deposition (CPPD) disease, periarticular calcifications are common in the elbow, wrist, and pelvis, but they coexist a majority of times with pathologic changes in the joint, in the form of either degenerative disease or chondrocalcinosis. These calcifications may occur either in the joint (intra-articular deposits) or around the joint (periarticular deposits) and may be related to both CPPD and hydroxyapatite crystal deposition. Calcification of a gouty tophus is an unusual finding and usually reflects a coexisting abnormality of calcium metabolism. Patients with sarcoidosis frequently demonstrate a reticular, or lacelike, pattern in the medullary cavity of the bones of the hand.

This patient was ultimately diagnosed with scleroderma.

Acromion Fracture

1. It is well protected by large muscles, so a considerable force is required to cause a fracture.

2. Lateral displacement of the scapula.

3. Two.

4. Concomitant fractures of the coracoid, ribs, and clavicle, and dislocation of the acromioclavicular joint. Axillary nerve.

Reference

Goss TP: The scapula: Coracoid, acromial, and avulsion fractures. Am J Orthop 25:106–115, 1996.

Comments

Scapular fractures are uncommon, accounting for about 1% of all fractures in the skeleton. A direct force causes most injuries to the scapula. Associated fractures of the ipsilateral ribs or clavicle occur in more than three fourths of cases. Fractures of the acromion process are considered rare injuries. They are also caused by direct trauma to the shoulder, although avulsion fractures owing to indirect forces and stress fractures may also occur. Most fractures involving the acromion process occur at the junction of the scapular spine and the acromion. These fractures are usually evident radiographically, particularly in the scapular Y view of the shoulder, and close inspection of the radiographs is all that is required for diagnosis. Occasionally, computed tomography may be required if adequate radiographs cannot be obtained. The majority of acromion fractures do not require surgical intervention, but when they are displaced, operative stabilization is needed to restore a normal functional result. Inferior displacement of the scapula from dislocation of the ipsilateral acromioclavicular joint can lead to an axillary nerve palsy.

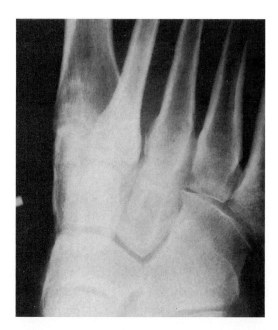
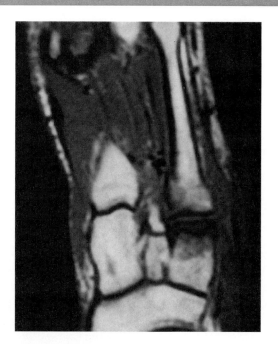
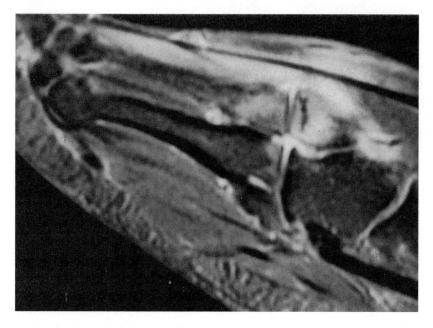

1. In the foot, where are the common sites for stress fractures?

2. Which imaging modality would you recommend first when evaluating a possible stress fracture of the foot in a high-caliber athlete?

3. When would you expect a stress fracture to be radiographically evident?

4. Regarding navicular stress fractures, what is the treatment of choice, and why?

Lateral Cuneiform Stress Fracture

1. Second and third metatarsals, calcaneus, talus, navicular, cuneiforms, and sesamoids.

2. Begin with radiographs. If these are normal, I would recommend magnetic resonance imaging (MRI) because it allows direct inspection of the marrow and provides high spatial resolution, capabilities that are not available with either computed tomography or bone scintigraphy.

3. Stress fractures become evident as early as 2 to 3 weeks after the onset of symptoms.

4. Complete non–weight bearing, because restricted activity is associated with a high incidence of nonunion.

Reference

Hamilton WC: Injuries of the ankle and foot. Emerg Med Clin North Am 2:361–389, 1984.

Comments

Most stress fractures are fatigue fractures caused by increased stresses on normal bone. They are common in the lower extremity, although cuneiform stress fractures are unusual. These fractures are significant in athletes who participate in sports that require running. Clinically, patients present with swelling of the dorsum of the foot and pain, which increases with activity and subsides with rest. A classic history is pain beginning within a few weeks of a change in the intensity of training. MRI is capable of demonstrating marrow edema in the medullary cavity before a stress fracture becomes evident on conventional radiographs. This finding is called a *stress phenomenon*. With continued exposure to the eliciting stress, a low signal intensity linear abnormality develops in the area of marrow edema extending to the cortex. This finding is a stress fracture. In my experience, cuneiform stress fractures are usually subchondral in location, in contradistinction to most navicular fractures, which occur in the sagittal plane and involve the middle and medial thirds of the bone. Navicular and cuneiform stress fractures may be extremely difficult to diagnose on conventional radiographs and almost always require cross-sectional imaging for accurate assessment.

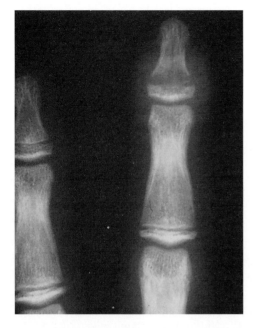

1. What is this injury called when it involves the toe?
2. What is the mechanism of injury?
3. What is important to know about a subungual hematoma? Where does it occur?
4. When the growth plate is involved, what fractures may occur?

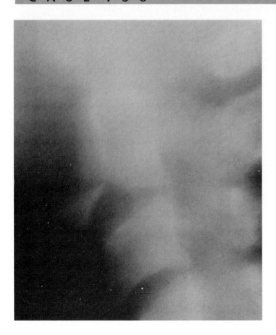

1. How many people suffer cord compression with this type of injury?
2. At what level is an articular pillar fracture likely to occur? What is the best way to diagnose this fracture?
3. What important complication may have occurred when a corner chip fracture caused by a hyperextension injury is no longer visible after reduction of the spine?
4. Most hyperextension fractures are stable. When are they unstable?

Distal Phalangeal Growth Plate Injuries

1. Stubbed toe syndrome.

2. Hyperflexion of the distal phalanx.

3. It should not be drained because it may create a direct communication to the bone. At the base of the nail.

4. Salter-Harris type 1 and 2 fractures.

Reference

Pinckney LE, Currarino G, Kennedy LA: The stubbed great toe: A cause of occult compound fracture and infection. Radiology 138:375-377, 1981.

Comments

Finger and toe injuries are common in children. A significant number of these injuries involve the growth plate. Fractures located at the epiphyseal plate of a distal phalanx, however, should be treated with great vigilance because many of these injuries actually represent unsuspected compound fractures. A thin layer of dermis separates the nail root from the dorsal periosteum of the base of the distal phalanx. An impaction injury may cause penetration of the nail root through this soft tissue and into the growth plate. Clinically, a small amount of bleeding from the nail fold or a more proximal laceration may occur at the time of injury, but this observation may escape detection once the cuticle has become edematous. Radiographically, a fracture through the epiphyseal plate may result in its widening or in displacement of the epiphysis from the metaphysis. Focal demineralization of the metaphysis may indicate the presence of osteomyelitis. Unchecked infection can progress quickly, destroying the bone and causing asymmetrical widening of the growth plate. Once advanced, an infection necessitates surgical débridement and prolonged antibiotic therapy. Premature closure of the epiphysis is a common sequela, producing a short distal phalanx.

Hyperextension C2 Fracture

1. About one fifth.

2. C6. Computed tomography (CT), because 60% of these fractures are missed on radiographs.

3. Entrapment into the disk space.

4. Isolated vertebral body fractures are stable. They become unstable when there is also a fracture of the posterior arch.

Reference

Berquist TH: Imaging of adult cervical spine trauma. Radiographics 8:667-694, 1988.

Comments

Hyperextension injury of the cervical spine is relatively common. It is caused by a superiorly directed force on the mandible or a posteriorly directed force on the forehead. The classic findings associated with this injury are prevertebral soft-tissue swelling, widening of the anterior disk space, and small triangular fracture from the anterior and inferior aspect of the vertebral body, which represents an avulsion fracture at the attachment site of the anterior longitudinal ligament. Most hyperextension fractures occur at C1 and C2. Posterior retrolisthesis at the level of ligamentous disruption can narrow the spinal canal and compress the cord. Vascular compromise can cause central cord syndrome.

When the majority of the force is absorbed by the posterior elements, one may see fractures involving the pedicle, lamina, articular pillar, and spinous process. Pillar fractures are notoriously difficult to diagnose on conventional radiographs. Patients may complain of radiculopathy, but a concomitant injury to the cord is unusual. These patients should have a CT examination of their cervical spine if a pillar fracture is not evident on initial radiographs. Fractures of the pedicle below C2 occur nearly exclusively with hyperextension injuries. Therefore, if you identify a fractured pedicle, increase your index of suspicion for other posterior arch fractures. The trick here is that 80% of pedicle fractures are missed on conventional radiographs, so you need to scrutinize the lateral and oblique radiographs very carefully.

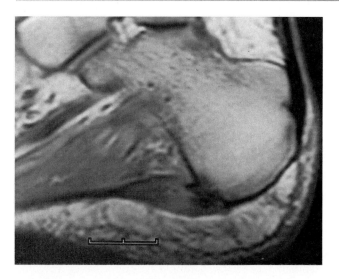
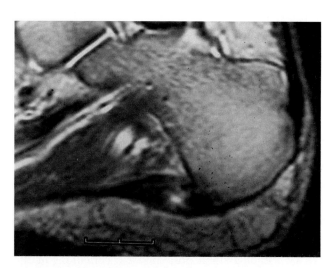

1. What is the diagnosis? What are some other causes of plantar heel pain?
2. Name the components of the plantar fascia. Which segments are affected by fasciitis?
3. What is the normal thickness of the plantar fascia?
4. What differentiates acute plantar fasciitis from chronic fasciitis?

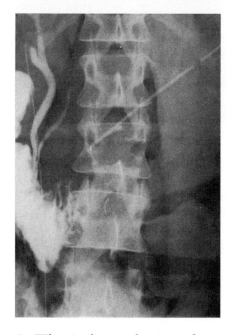
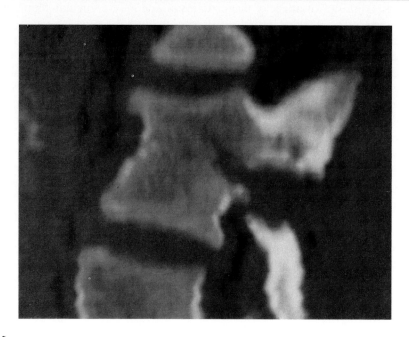

1. What is the mechanism of injury?
2. Is this considered a stable or an unstable injury acutely?
3. Is this a common injury?
4. Which area is most likely to be involved?

Plantar Fasciitis

1. Acute plantar fasciitis. Tarsal tunnel syndrome, stress fractures, and plantar fascia rupture.

2. Medial, central, and lateral cords. The central cord is nearly always affected, but the lateral cord may be involved as well.

3. The normal thickness is between 3.2 mm and 3.4 mm.

4. The presence of edema in and about the aponeurosis.

References

Berkowitz JF, Kier R, Rudicel S: Plantar fasciitis: MR imaging. Radiology 179:665–667, 1991.

Yu JS: Pathologic and post-operative conditions of the plantar fascia: Review of MR imaging appearances. Skeletal Radiol 29:491–501, 2000.

Comments

Plantar fasciitis is a painful condition that has been attributed to repeated mechanical stresses that cause chronic microtears of the calcaneal attachment of the plantar aponeurosis. Plantar fasciitis is a straightforward diagnosis, but the advantage of magnetic resonance imaging over other imaging modalities is the ability to differentiate an acute exacerbation from occurrences that are less acute. The hallmark of plantar fasciitis is marked thickening (typically a twofold to threefold increase) of the calcaneal attachment of the central cord of the plantar aponeurosis. When a patient is experiencing acute focal pain, the insertion will demonstrate signal alterations in the aponeurosis consistent with edema. Perifascial edema causes indistinctness of the margins of the fascia. Edema in the subcutaneous fat is usually evident as well. Inversion recovery imaging may be more sensitive to changes in the adjacent bone marrow than is conventional spin-echo imaging, and it is useful in excluding stress fractures. When the condition is more chronic, or if the patient responds to a course of conservative therapy, regional soft-tissue edema will diminish and the signal alterations in the fascia will dissipate. In the majority of patients with chronic plantar fasciitis, an enthesophyte will develop at the enthesis of the plantar fascia after a few months.

Chance Fracture (L2)

1. Abrupt deceleration against an automobile seat belt.

2. Acutely, this fracture is considered unstable. Pure osseous fractures have excellent healing potential, and long-term stability is likely, but pure ligamentous injuries have a low healing potential and a high risk of residual instability.

3. No, but it is not uncommon either, because it accounts for about 10% of all major fractures of the spine.

4. The fractures occur between T12 and L4, with 50% occurring at L2, L3, and L4.

Reference

Ashman CJ, Yu JS, Chung CB: The Chance fracture: Anteroposterior radiographic signs. Emerg Radiol 4:320–325, 1997.

Comments

The Chance fracture was initially described as a horizontal fracture that started in the spinous process and neural arch, extended into the vertebral body, and exited through the superior end plate anterior to the neural foramen. Since then, three additional patterns have been described. These range from purely ligamentous injuries to fractures that involve all three columns of the spine. Compression of the vertebral body is not a major finding. The mechanism of injury is related to the anterior position of the fulcrum of force during forced flexion of the torso. The restraint of a lap seat belt results in only tensile forces on the spine, so the primary injury is distraction.

A good lateral view generally is diagnostic, but often this cannot be obtained in a patient who has sustained multiple trauma. Computed tomography through the area of interest with sagittal reformatted images may be helpful, but the diagnosis can be achieved through careful inspection of an anteroposterior radiograph of the thoracolumbar spine. Pertinent observations include increased interspinal distance (empty hole sign), splitting of the pedicle, fracture of the spinous process, fracture of the lamina, widening of the disk space or facet joints, and widening of the intercostal space.

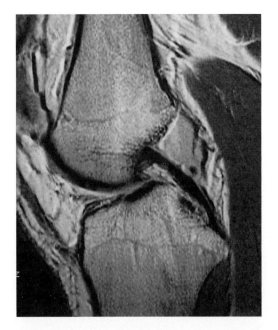 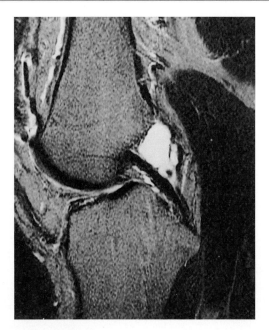

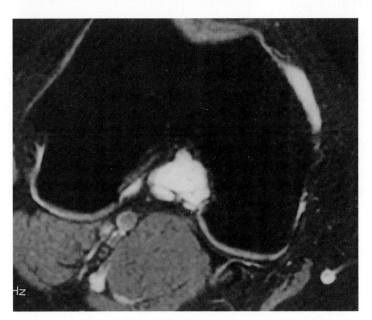

1. What are some conditions that can cause this appearance?

2. Can intra-articular ganglion cysts cause osseous erosion? Which ones can?

3. Histologically, what is a ganglion cyst?

4. What is the most common presentation of a patient with an intra-articular ganglion cyst?

Cruciate Ganglion Cyst

1. Cruciate ganglion cyst, meniscal cyst, synovial cyst.

2. Yes, those that arise from the posterior cruciate ligament.

3. Cystic cavities lined by cells that are not of true synovial origin containing clear mucinous fluid.

4. Pain and limitation of the range of motion.

Reference

Recht MP, Applegate G, Kaplan P, et al: The MR appearance of cruciate ganglion cysts: A report of 16 cases. Skeletal Radiol 23:597–600, 1994.

Comments

Extra-articular cysts arising about the knee joint are common and likely represent popliteal cysts, meniscal cysts, and ganglion cysts. Intra-articular cysts, on the other hand, are uncommon and most likely represent either meniscal cysts or ganglion cysts. A cruciate ganglion cyst is an unusual entity that presents as a well-defined, multilocular lesion arising from either the posterior or the anterior cruciate ligament. On T1W images, these cysts vary from hypointense to slightly hyperintense with respect to the signal intensity of muscle. On T2W images, the majority of cysts demonstrate homogeneously high signal intensity, although hemorrhage may alter the signal characteristics of a particular lesion. The differential diagnosis is limited. Trapped joint effusion can be eliminated owing to the multilocular nature of the majority of posterior cruciate ligament lesions and the fusiform appearance of anterior cruciate ligament lesions. Occasionally, a large intra-articular meniscal cyst arising from the posterior horn of either meniscus can mimic this ganglion cyst, but the presence of a large meniscal tear should be evident.

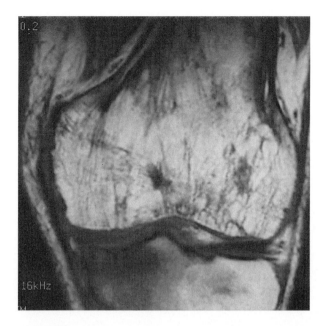

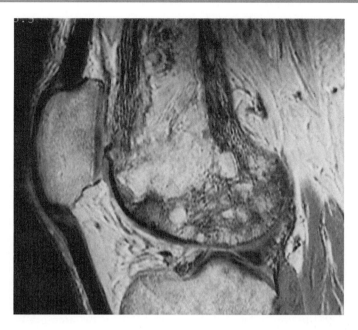

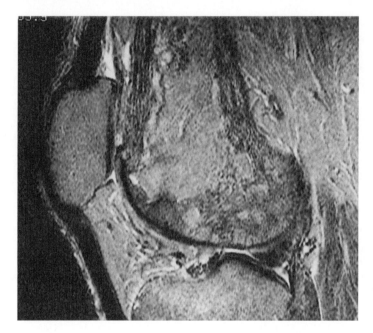

1. What caused the changes in this patient's femur?

2. What does the term *mosaic pattern* refer to in this disease?

3. What is characteristic about osteoporosis circumscripta?

4. If this patient has a sudden rise in the serum alkaline phosphatase level, what does it indicate?

Paget's Disease

1. Paget's disease.

2. A patternless arrangement of coarsened and enlarged osseous trabeculae.

3. It generally involves only the outer table of the skull.

4. Sarcomatous degeneration.

Reference

Griffiths HJ: Radiology of Paget's disease. Curr Opin Radiol 4:124–128, 1992.

Comments

This case is challenging without the aid of a corresponding radiograph. However, if you inspect the magnetic resonance imaging findings closely, you'll quickly recognize that they parallel those that you would expect to find on a radiograph. Paget's disease is characterized by destruction of bone (lytic phase) followed by attempts at repair (reparative phase). The lytic phase of the disease may predominate early in the disease process, but more frequently there is a combination of destruction and repair. The osteosclerotic phase is characterized by osteoblastic activity. In the quiescent phase, bone resorption and cellular activity are absent. The magnetic resonance imaging appearance of Paget's disease depends on the phase of the disease and the extent of reparative bone. If repair is limited, lysis manifested by bone marrow edema is a dominant finding. During this phase of the disease, it may be difficult to exclude a neoplastic process. As the disease progresses, regions of diminished signal intensity within the medullary cavity reflect bone repair. Coarsened trabeculae become a conspicuous network of thick, linear, low signal intensity bands. Although thickened, the cortex appears irregular and laminated, demonstrating signal intensities on T1W and T2W images that are considerably higher than those of normal cortex. This magnetic resonance imaging finding correlates with the radiographic observation that the thickened cortex in pagetoid bone appears less dense and often mottled. When Paget's disease is widely disseminated, the serum alkaline phosphatase level may be elevated. An acute elevation, however, heralds malignant transformation.

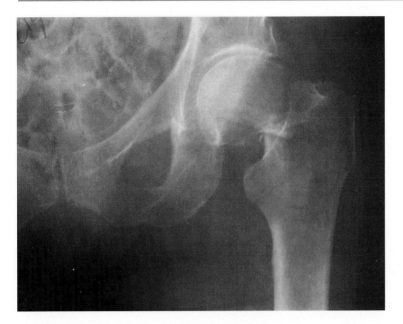

1. Which type of femur fracture has the highest risk of developing avascular necrosis (AVN)?

2. What is Garden's classification?

3. What vessels supply the femoral head?

4. Does this patient have a high risk for developing AVN of the femoral head? Why?

Subcapital Femur Fracture

1. Subcapital femur fractures.

2. The most common classification for intracapsular hip fractures. Garden I, incomplete or impacted fracture; Garden II, complete fracture without displacement; Garden III, complete fracture with varus angulation; and Garden IV, complete fracture with total displacement.

3. Medial and lateral epiphyseal arteries and the artery of the ligamentum teres.

4. Yes. The more angulated the fracture, the more likely it is that AVN will develop.

Reference

Yu JS: Hip and femur trauma. Imaging of trauma to the extremities. Semin Musculoskeletal Radiol 4:205–220, 2000.

Comments

Subcapital fractures occur just distal to the articular margin of the femoral head. Fractures that occur through the neck of the femur are referred to as *transcervical* fractures, and those that occur at the junction of the neck and the shaft are referred to as *basocervical* fractures. Two important potential complications of subcapital fractures are fracture nonunion and AVN of the femoral head. The more proximal the fracture line, the greater the incidence of both complications. The femoral head is supplied by three terminal arterial sources. The main arterial supply of the adult femoral head originates from the medial and lateral femoral circumflex arteries, which may arise from either the femoral artery or the deep femoral artery. At the base of the femoral neck, terminal branches of the medial circumflex artery (medial epiphyseal artery) and the lateral circumflex artery (lateral epiphyseal artery) converge to form a vascular ring that supplies numerous ascending cervical arterial vessels. The artery of the ligamentum teres also contributes blood supply to the femoral head epiphyseal region. The leading factors contributing to the development of AVN of the femoral head are disruption of the epiphyseal arteries or the vessels that supply these terminal vessels and unstable reduction of a fracture. Angulated and displaced neck fractures tether these end arteries, disrupting the blood supply.

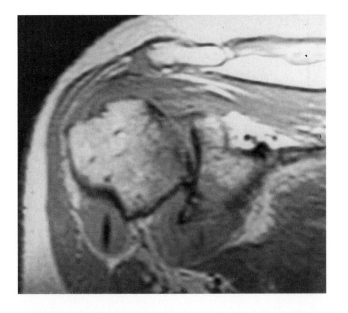
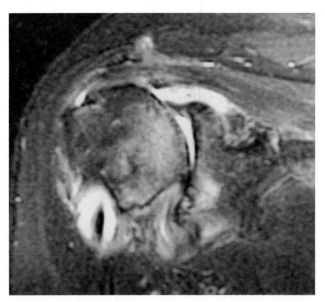
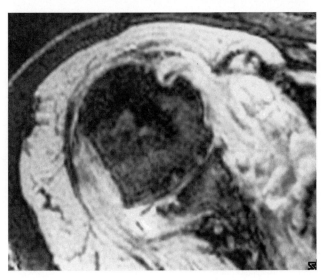

1. List the diagnostic considerations in this patient.

2. Aspiration of the joint is likely to reveal what findings? How often does it occur in the absence of radiographically detectable calcification?

3. What pathologic cascade causes the structural damage?

4. What is mixed calcium phosphate crystal deposition disease?

Milwaukee Shoulder Syndrome

1. Crystal deposition arthropathies, secondary osteoarthritis, infection, and neuropathic arthropathy.

2. Calcium hydroxyapatite (HA) crystals. In about 80% of cases.

3. HA crystals are released into the synovial fluid, which becomes engulfed by fixed macrophage-like synovial cells that release the enzymes collagenase and protease, which attack the periarticular tissues, including the rotator cuff, which destabilizes the joint, which causes progressive joint destruction, which releases more crystals into the fluid.

4. Presence of both HA and calcium pyrophosphate dihydrate crystals in the joint.

Reference

Nguyen VD: Rapid destructive arthritis of the shoulder. Skeletal Radiol 25:107–112, 1996.

Comments

Capsular, tendinous, ligamentous, and bursal calcification are common in patients with HA crystal deposition disease. Initially, the disease may cause minimal or no symptoms, but it can progress to tenderness, swelling, and restricted motion. Milwaukee shoulder syndrome refers to structural damage caused by deposition of HA crystals in the shoulder. Radiographic findings include loss of joint space, destruction of bone, subchondral sclerosis, intra-articular debris, and joint disorganization and deformity. Subchondral cyst formation and osteophytosis are relatively uncommon. Rotator cuff tears result in the superior migration of the humeral head, which often contacts the inferior surface of the acromion, resulting in mechanical erosive changes from direct bone-to-bone contact. The magnetic resonance imaging features of this condition parallel those findings that are evident radiographically. Magnetic resonance imaging has the added advantage of characterizing the damage to the periarticular soft tissues. In this patient, there was a full-thickness rotator cuff tear, damaged articular hyaline cartilage, extensive labrum tears, synovitis, and periarticular marrow edema in addition to the expected structural damage described earlier.

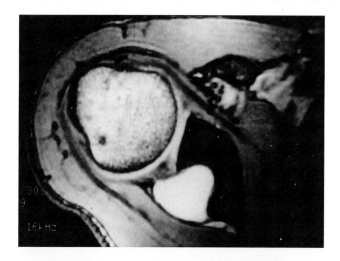

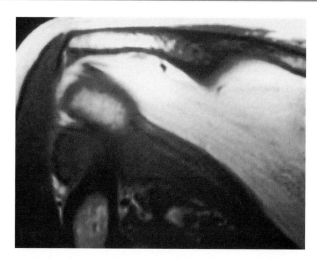

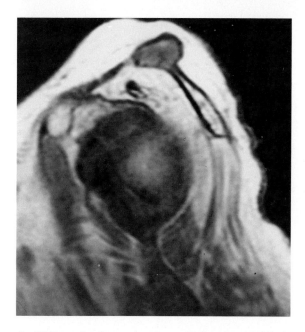

1. Where is the epicenter of this lesion if the supraspinatus muscle is normal?

2. When assessing scapular fractures, what is a critical observation to include in your report?

3. Is there anything you can do to relieve the nerve compression before definitive treatment is performed?

4. What other common neuropathy may occur in the shoulder?

Suprascapular Nerve Entrapment

1. Below the spinoglenoid notch.

2. Extension of a fracture line to the suprascapular notch.

3. Yes, aspiration of the cyst.

4. Axillary nerve compression (quadrilateral space syndrome).

Reference

Fritz RC, Helms CA, Steinbach LS, Genant HK: Suprascapular nerve entrapment: Evaluation with MR imaging. Radiology 182:437–444, 1992.

Comments

The suprascapular nerve is a mixed motor and sensory nerve that contains pain fibers to the shoulder and provides the motor supply to the supraspinatus and infraspinatus muscles of the rotator cuff. Some common causes of suprascapular nerve entrapment are a suprascapular notch ganglion, a perilabrum cyst, and tumors. If the nerve is injured or entrapped, the location of insult determines if both muscles are affected or if only the infraspinatus muscle is affected. The typical appearance of subacute muscle denervation is high signal intensity on T2W images in the affected muscle. The altered signal intensity in the muscle reflects an increase in the extracellular water space, which increases the T1 and T2 relaxation times. The total water content of the muscle is only minimally increased—a finding attributed to simultaneous shrinking of the myoplasm. These changes may be detected as early as 2 weeks from the time of injury or entrapment, and the outcome depends on the promptness of treatment. If the nerve entrapment is not treated, there is usually progression to irreversible fatty change and atrophy of the muscle. On T1W images, this is reflected by an increase in high signal intensity tissue between the muscle fibers, producing a striated appearance in the muscle.

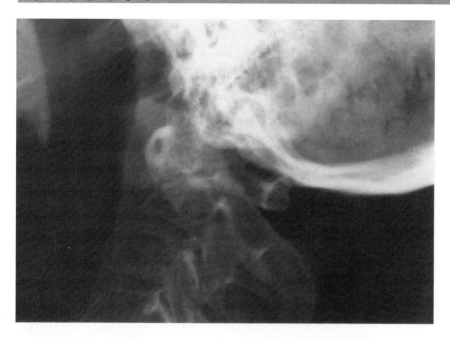

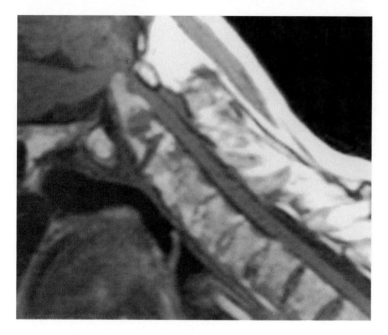

1. Identify the process that is occurring at the atlantoaxial joint.

2. What symptoms would you expect?

3. Why is this not basilar invagination?

4. Define atlantoaxial subluxation. On average, when do patients with rheumatoid arthritis (RA) become symptomatic?

Rheumatoid Arthritis (Cranial Settling)

1. Cranial settling.

2. Pain is the most common symptom, exacerbated by neck motion. Paresthesias or weakness of both upper and lower extremities, loss of deep tendon reflexes, quadriparesis, and cord compression are other symptoms.

3. The tip of the dens is below McRae's line.

4. Predental space exceeds 2.5 mm. At about 9 mm.

Reference

Zeidman SM, Ducker TB: Rheumatoid arthritis. Neuroanatomy, compression, and grading of deficits. Spine 19:2259-2266, 1994.

Comments

Involvement of the cervical spine occurs in nearly 70% of patients with long-standing RA. Approximately one third of these patients develop subluxation in the anterior, posterior, lateral, or transaxial directions. Fortunately, only a small percentage of these patients develop neurologic symptoms. However, once neurologic symptoms occur, compressive myelopathy may progress rapidly.

Anterior atlantoaxial subluxation is characterized by anterior displacement of the atlas, causing an increased space between the dens and the anterior arch of C1. When the odontoid process and the transverse ligaments are destroyed, the atlas may also shift in a posterior direction. Destruction of the lateral masses may result in cranial settling or lateral subluxation (torticollis) if the erosion is asymmetrical. This patient clearly shows evidence of cranial settling. Cranial settling is a process that is characterized by inferior migration of the atlas relative to the odontoid process, caused by destruction of both lateral masses of C1 and by collapse of the occipitoatlantal and atlantoaxial articulations. A clue to the diagnosis of cranial settling is recognition that the anterior arch of C1 (which normally articulates with the odontoid process) articulates with the base of the odontoid or the body of C2. On magnetic resonance images, pannus frequently demonstrates low signal intensity on both T1W and T2W images, owing in part to deposition of hemosiderin in the hypertrophied synovium. High signal intensity tissue on T2W images may be related to either active pannus or granulation tissue caused by chronic friction from the instability.

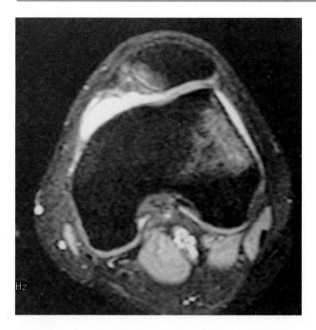

1. What injury did this patient have at one time? Name the different types of dislocations.
2. When you observe this contusion pattern, what other abnormality should you look for?
3. What must be present for an intra-articular dislocation to occur?
4. How do superior dislocations occur, and in whom?

Lateral Patellar Dislocation

1. Lateral patellar dislocation. Lateral, medial, superior, and intra-articular patellar dislocations.

2. Osteochondral defects of either the patella or the lateral femoral condyle.

3. A complete quadriceps tendon tear.

4. They occur in the elderly population when the patella becomes locked on an anterior femoral osteophyte during hyperextension of the knee.

Reference

Yu JS, Cook PA: Magnetic resonance imaging (MRI) of the knee: A pattern approach for evaluating bone marrow edema. Crit Rev Diagn Imaging 37:261–303, 1996.

Comments

True patellar dislocations are relatively less common than is subluxation of the patella; they are caused by tracking abnormalities of the extensor mechanism. A lateral patellar dislocation is the most common type of patellar dislocation and occurs when there is forced internal rotation of the femur on a fixed, externally rotated tibia with the knee in flexion. The pull of the quadriceps muscles on the patella causes it to displace out of the trochlea. When there is significant displacement, the medial retinaculum tears, which allows impaction between the medial patellar facet and the lateral surface of the lateral femoral condyle. If this occurs with sufficient force to produce bone contusions, a characteristic "kissing" bone contusion pattern is created, as demonstrated by this patient. Magnetic resonance imaging has played an important role in identifying unsuspected osteochondral or pure chondral defects of the hyaline cartilage of the patella or trochlea in patients who have persistent anterior knee pain after a dislocation of the patella.

Challenge

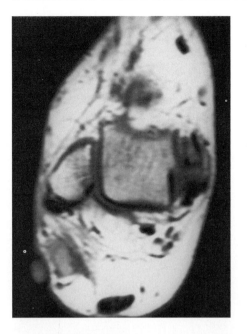 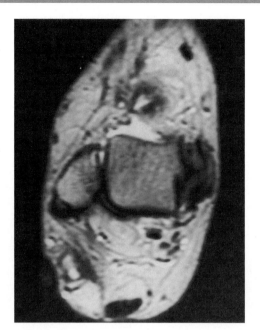

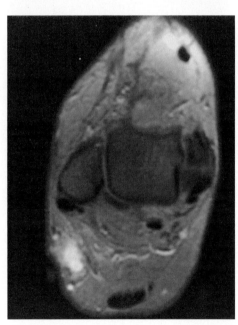

1. What is the most likely diagnosis?

2. How does a schwannoma differ from a neurofibroma?

3. Can these lesions be differentiated based on their magnetic resonance imaging characteristics?

4. How are schwannomas classified histologically?

Peripheral Schwannoma

1. A peripheral schwannoma of the sural nerve.

2. Tissue of origin. Schwannoma has a nerve sheath origin; neurofibroma has a nerve root or peripheral nerve origin.

3. For solitary lesions, this may be difficult to do. Cysts and hemorrhage favor a schwannoma. Low signal on T2W favors neurofibroma.

4. Antoni type A (cell rich and composed of compact bundles of fibrillated cells) and Antoni type B (loosely textured stroma with microcystic degeneration with mucin).

Reference

Demachi H, Takashima T, Kadoya M, et al: MR imaging of spinal neurinomas with pathologic correlation. J Comput Assist Tomogr 14:250–254, 1990.

Comments

The principal observation in this case is a mass in the posterolateral aspect of the ankle, along the distribution of the sural nerve. The key to the diagnosis is close scrutiny of the signal characteristics of the lesion demonstrated on the T2W and fat-saturated T1W post–gadolinium administration images. At first inspection, on the basis of the T2W image, you may want to entertain the possibility of a cystic mass, such as a ganglion, a hematoma, or maybe even a varix. However, the homogeneous enhancement of the lesion excludes all these possibilities, and a neural tumor remains the only plausible diagnosis.

A schwannoma (also referred to as a neuroma, a neurilemoma, or a peripheral fibroblastoma) is a neural tumor of nerve sheath origin that arises along nerve roots or peripheral nerves. It is usually solitary but may be multiple in patients with neurofibromatosis. On magnetic resonance imaging, these lesions appear isointense to hypointense to muscle on T1W images and hyperintense on T2W images (sometimes marked), and the images are enhanced with administration of intravenous contrast. These tumors frequently have cystic and hemorrhagic components (both demonstrated in this case) in addition to the solid component. Neurofibromas, on the other hand, are uniformly solid, although central areas of decreased signal intensity on T2W images indicate a more collagenous stroma.

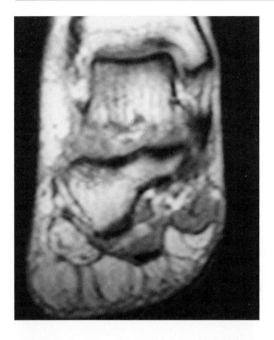
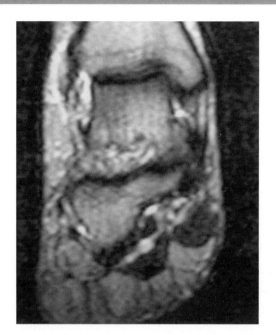
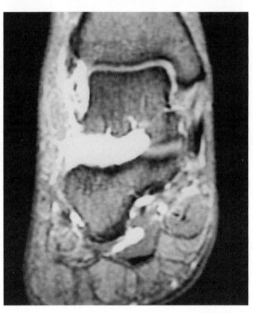

1. What is the most common cause of this disorder?

2. Are the magnetic resonance imaging findings in this patient consistent with this diagnosis? What is the tissue that is enhanced?

3. What other soft-tissue injuries are commonly seen in patients with this syndrome?

4. If contrast is injected into the posterior subtalar joint, what will you see if the interosseous ligament is disrupted?

Sinus Tarsi Syndrome

1. Trauma (inversion of the ankle) causing tears of one or both ligaments (cervical and interosseous) of the sinus tarsi.

2. Yes. Hypertrophied synovium.

3. Tears of the anterior talofibular and calcaneofibular ligaments and injuries of the peroneal tendons.

4. Extravasation of contrast into the sinus tarsi.

Reference

Beltran J: Sinus tarsi syndrome. Magn Reson Imaging Clin N Am 2:59-65, 1994.

Comments

The sinus tarsi is a funnel-shaped space between the talus and the calcaneus, its narrow opening located just posterior to the middle subtalar joint and its wider lateral opening seen just superior to the anterior calcaneal process. The artery of the tarsal canal, the end nerves, the ligaments (interosseous and cervical), and the medial fibers of the inferior extensor retinaculum are found within this space. The ligaments of the sinus tarsi contribute to hindfoot stabilization. Sinus tarsi syndrome is a painful condition characterized by pain over the lateral aspect of the sinus tarsi, often accompanied by sensations of instability and weakness. In nearly 75% of cases, this syndrome is caused by disruption of the interosseous ligaments, the cervical ligaments, or both; it is acquired during an inversion injury. This can lead to the development of synovial hyperplasia, which then becomes a space-occupying process in the sinus tarsi. On magnetic resonance images, the condition has a characteristic appearance. Poor definition of the ligaments, edema in the soft tissues in the sinus tarsi, and marked enhancement of hypertrophic synovium after administration of intravenous gadolinium are typical findings. Other conditions can cause sinus tarsi syndrome, however; these include synovial inflammatory diseases such as rheumatoid arthritis and gout, peroneal nerve entrapment, ganglion cysts, tumors, and osteoarthritis.

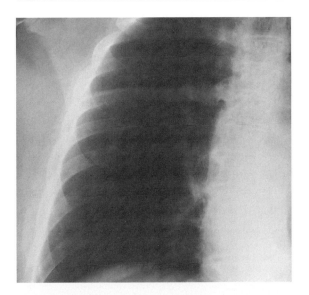
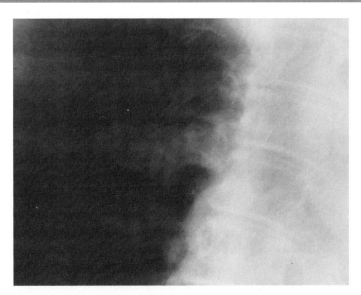
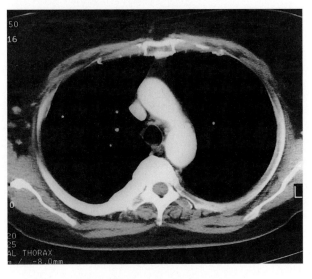

1. What is the differential diagnosis?

2. Why is metastasis unlikely?

3. Can ankylosis of the costovertebral joint occur in this condition?

4. List some characteristic findings of diffuse idiopathic skeletal hyperostosis (DISH) in the thoracic spine.

C A S E 1 6 8

Rib Hyperostosis Associated with DISH

1. Hyperostosis of the rib associated with DISH, melorheostosis, and Paget's disease.

2. It is not a consideration because of the involvement of both vertebral body and rib and the intervening costovertebral joint.

3. Yes.

4. Ossification along the anterolateral aspect of the vertebral body and disk, calcification of the intervertebral disks, elongation and hyperostosis of spinous processes, and ossification of the interspinous ligaments.

Reference

Huang GS, Park YH, Taylor JAM, et al: Hyperostosis of ribs: Association with vertebral ossification. J Rheumatol 20:2073–2076, 1993.

Comments

Proliferative bone changes in the axial skeleton producing rib hyperostosis are common in disorders that principally affect the spine. They are most commonly associated with DISH, accounting for more than 21% of cases of rib hyperostosis, whereas 10% of cases are associated with ankylosing spondylitis and 7% of cases are associated with quadriplegia. The mechanism that causes cortical thickening and sclerosis of ribs is unknown but is hypothesized to be a stress-related phenomenon or a consequence of the propensity for ossification in these spinal disorders. The radiographic features of rib hyperostosis are characterized by cortical thickening and dense bone sclerosis involving the posteromedial portion of a rib. The head of the rib may enlarge and expand anteriorly as a result of metaplastic ossification of the surrounding ligaments at the costovertebral joint and subligamentous connective tissue, mimicking the changes of Paget's disease. Nearly 75% of cases affect only one rib; about 20% involve two levels and 5% involve three levels, but these do not occur in contiguous ribs. The majority of hyperostosis occurs between the 5th and 10th ribs. Costovertebral excrescences frequently develop at the level of rib hyperostosis, which limits motion of the adjacent costovertebral joints. When this condition is suspected, computed tomography is advocated for further evaluation.

In the differential, melorheostosis is a consideration, but it is a rare condition and not as likely if the characteristic findings of DISH are evident in the spine. Paget's disease is also rarely seen in the ribs.

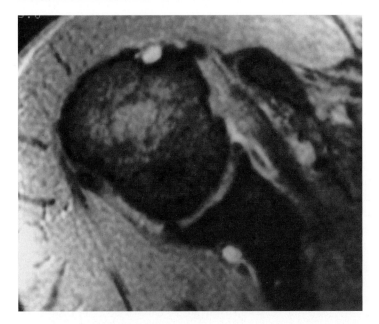

1. Where are the two tendinous attachments of the biceps brachii muscle?

2. List the restraints of the tendon of the long head of the biceps.

3. What are the two types of tendinous dislocations? Which is more common?

4. What is a Buford complex?

Medial Dislocation of the Biceps Tendon

1. The short head—tip of the coracoid process adjacent to the coracobrachialis muscle. The long head—superior rim of the glenoid at the bicipital tubercle and the glenoid labrum.

2. The coracohumeral ligament, superior glenohumeral ligament, and transverse humeral ligament, with contributions from the subscapularis tendon.

3. Extra-articular—anteromedial displacement of the tendon associated with an intact subscapularis muscle and tendon; intra-articular—a defect in the subscapularis attachment on the lesser tuberosity allowing displacement of the tendon into the glenohumeral joint. Extra-articular.

4. Congenital absence of the anterosuperior labrum with a cordlike middle glenohumeral ligament.

Reference

Cervilla V, Schweitzer ME, Ho C, et al: Medial dislocation of the biceps brachii tendon: Appearance at MR imaging. Radiology 180:523-526, 1991.

Comments

Degenerative changes in the rotator cuff tendons may sometimes cause a dislocation of the tendon of the long head of the biceps brachii muscle. Impingement can be an important factor, causing disruption of the coracohumeral ligament, one of the intra-articular restraints of the biceps tendon, and the anterior fibers of the supraspinatus tendon. This allows the biceps tendon to dislocate out of the bicipital groove. Clinically, patients complain of shoulder pain or of a snapping sensation in the shoulder during flexion and rotation of the elbow. Dislocation of the biceps tendon is shown best on axial magnetic resonance imaging. A normal tendon sits within the bicipital groove as either an ovoid or a semilunar low signal intensity structure. In this case, the tendon has displaced medially, coming to rest anterior to the lesser tuberosity. The bicipital groove is empty ("empty groove" sign). When evaluating a potential tendon dislocation, it is critical to take note of the integrity of the transverse humeral ligament and the subscapularis tendon to correctly classify the biceps tendon dislocation. This can be difficult because the tendon may come to rest in a number of locations from the lesser tuberosity to the anterior glenoid. Occasionally, a dislocated tendon mimics an anterior labrum tear or a Buford complex.

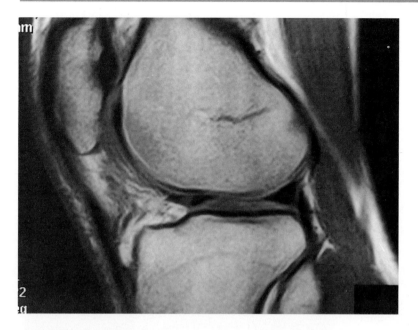

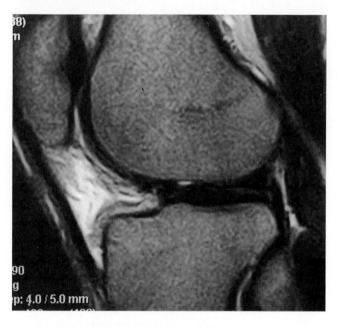

1. List the differential diagnosis.
2. How would you expect this patient to present?
3. Is there an association between this disorder and osteoarthritis?
4. In chronic cases, what tissues or substances affect the magnetic resonance imaging appearance?

Hoffa's Disease

1. Hoffa's disease, intracapsular chondroma, complex meniscal cyst, complex synovial cyst.

2. Pain in the anterior aspect of the knee, exacerbated by extension.

3. Yes, owing to synovial trapping.

4. Fibrin and hemosiderin deposition.

Reference

Jacobson JA, Lenchik L, Ruhoy MK, et al: MR imaging of the infrapatellar fat pad of Hoffa. Radiographics 17:675–691, 1997.

Comments

The infrapatellar fat pad of Hoffa is a triangular fat compartment in the anterior aspect of the knee. Hoffa's disease is a painful condition caused by one acute traumatic episode or repetitive trauma to the anterior knee that produces hemorrhage and necrosis in the fat pad. The inflamed fat pad becomes hypertrophied, further predisposing it to traumatic impingement between the femur and the tibia. Hoffa's syndrome is an entity similar to Hoffa's disease but occurs in the absence of known trauma. It is generally accepted that joint space narrowing secondary to degenerative joint disease, such as osteoarthritis, contributes to the development of the syndrome when there is synovial trapping. Clinically, patients complain of long-standing pain in the anterior compartment of the knee. Swelling may be evident on both sides of the patellar tendon. Forced extension exacerbates the pain owing to increased pressure on the fat pad. Infrapatellar bursitis may accompany the disease process.

The diagnosis is conspicuous on magnetic resonance imaging. Patients with Hoffa's disease demonstrate areas of intense edema within the infrapatellar fat pad during the acute phase of the disease. Bowing of the patellar tendon from mass effect may be evident. When the condition is chronic or subacute, fibrin and hemosiderin depositions affect the signal intensity in the fat, producing regions of low signal intensity on T1W and T2W images.

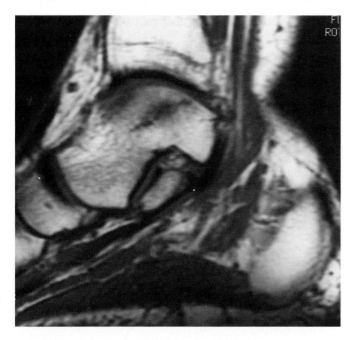 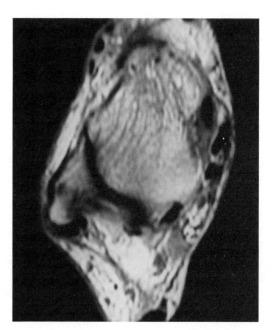

1. How do you think this patient presented?
2. Where is the transverse interfascicular septum, and what does it separate?
3. List some causes of tarsal tunnel syndrome.
4. How is tarsal tunnel syndrome treated?

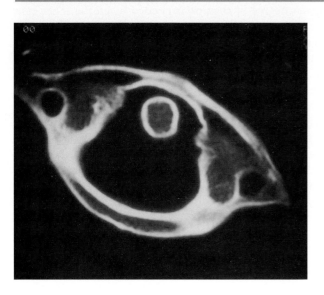 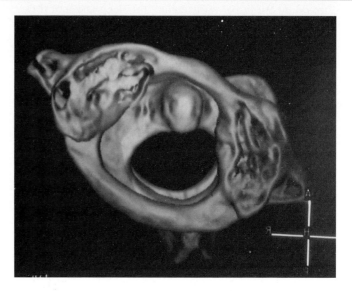

1. What are some common causes of C1 subluxation?
2. What is the most common type of rotary fixation of C1? What type does this patient have?
3. How do you differentiate rotary fixation from torticollis, and what imaging technique would you recommend?
4. How do you determine rotary subluxation radiographically?

Tarsal Tunnel Syndrome

1. With tarsal tunnel syndrome.

2. Connective tissue band between the medial surface of the calcaneus and the abductor hallucis muscle. Medial and lateral plantar nerves (branches of posterior tibial nerve).

3. Trauma, neoplasms, ganglions or other cysts, varicose veins, muscle anomalies, taut flexor retinaculum, tenosynovitis, mass or hypertrophy of abductor hallucis muscle, and neuroarthropathy.

4. Surgical decompression of the flexor retinaculum or resection of the causative lesion.

References

O'Malley GM, Lambdin CS, McCleary GS: Tarsal tunnel syndrome. Orthopedics 8:758-760, 1985.

Zeiss J, Ebraheim N, Rusin J: Magnetic resonance imaging in the diagnosis of tarsal tunnel syndrome. Case report. Clin Imaging 14:123-126, 1990.

Comments

The tarsal tunnel is a space in the foot that contains the medial tendons of the ankle, the posterior tibial nerve, and the medial vascular structures. The tunnel extends from the level of the medial malleolus to the tarsal navicular. The floor is composed of the tibia, the talus, the sustentaculum tali, and the calcaneus. Its roof is formed by the flexor retinaculum, the deep fascia of the lower extremity, and the abductor hallucis muscle. The tendons of the posterior tibial, flexor digitorum longus, and flexor hallucis longus muscles are separated from the neurovascular bundle by fibrous septation. The septa are attached to the neurovascular bundle, causing it to be relatively immobile. The posterior tibial nerve, accompanied by an artery and a vein, bifurcates into the medial and lateral plantar nerves beneath the flexor retinaculum, and these nerves are separated by the transverse interfascicular septum. Tarsal tunnel syndrome is an entrapment neuropathy of the posterior tibial nerve or one of its branches. Pain, paresthesia, sensory deficits, and weakness are characteristic symptoms of this syndrome. Magnetic resonance imaging is the preferred method for diagnosing this condition because this imaging technique allows unimpeded visualization of the tarsal tunnel and its contents. The cause of the syndrome in this patient was an anomalous accessory flexor digitorum longus muscle.

Atlantoaxial Rotary Subluxation

1. Inflammatory arthropathies such as rheumatoid arthritis, psoriasis, and ankylosing spondylitis; retropharyngeal infection; Behçet's syndrome; congenital anomalies; and trauma.

2. Type 1. Type 1.

3. Look for fixed C1 and C2 motion when the cervical spine is rotated. Computed tomography.

4. Using odontoid projections, have the patient tilt her or his head toward one ear and then toward the other. If the odontoid process remains positioned more closely toward the same lateral mass on both views, rotary subluxation is likely.

Reference

Fielding JW, Hawkins RJ: Atlanto-axial rotary fixation. J Bone Joint Surg Am 59:37-44, 1977.

Comments

Traumatic dislocation of the C1 vertebra is rare. The transverse ligament is the primary stabilizer that maintains the anatomic alignment of the atlas to the axis. Subluxation of the C1 vertebra on C2 can occur, however, when there is a fracture of the odontoid process or an avulsion of the transverse ligament. About 65 degrees of rotation is required to induce rotary fixation of C1 when these two structures are intact; however, a lesser degree of rotation is needed when the transverse ligament is ruptured. In a rotary fixation, the C1 and C2 vertebrae maintain a constant relationship when the spine is rotated, in contradistinction to the independent motion of these two vertebral bodies depicted in normal spines. The Fielding-Hawkins classification describes four types of rotary fixation. Type 1—rotary fixation without anterior subluxation; type 2—rotary fixation with 3 to 5 mm of atlantoaxial subluxation; type 3—rotary fixation with greater than 5 mm of atlantoaxial subluxation; and type 4—rotary fixation with posterior atlantoaxial subluxation.

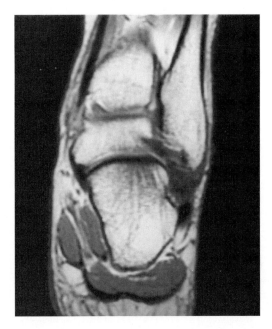 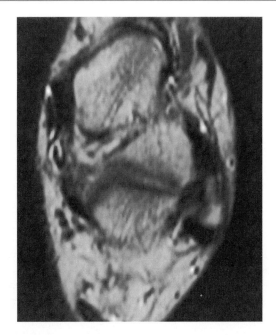

1. What is the etiology of this patient's chronic ankle pain?
2. Where is the anterolateral compartment of the ankle?
3. What is a "meniscoid" lesion?
4. Can interposition of an accessory fascicle of the anterior tibiofibular ligament cause similar symptoms?

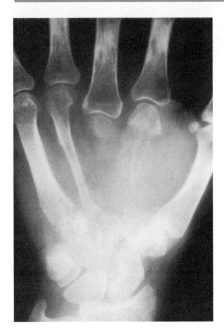

1. List your differential diagnosis.
2. Does the appearance of the fourth metacarpal bone help narrow these considerations?
3. What is Dupuytren's contracture, and what associations does it have?
4. Is this pathologic process similar to that of Gorham's disease?

Lateral Impingement Syndrome of the Ankle

1. Lateral impingement syndrome.

2. A space limited by the anterolateral talus, the antero-medial fibula, the calcaneofibular ligament, the anterolateral tibia, and the anterior talofibular ligament.

3. This is a descriptive term for hypertrophic synovial scar tissue in the anterolateral compartment (it mimics the appearance of a meniscus when viewed at surgery).

4. Yes.

References

Hauger O, Moinard M, Lasalarie JC, et al: Anterolateral compartment of the ankle in the lateral impingement syndrome: Appearance on CT arthrography. AJR Am J Roentgenol 173:685-690, 1999.

Long D, Yu JS, Vitellas K: The ankle joint: Imaging strategies in the evaluation of ligamentous injuries. Crit Rev Diagn Imaging 39:393-445, 1998.

Comments

Chronic pain in patients who have suffered trauma to the ankle is a common phenomenon, particularly in athletes. The causes are diverse and can be related to pathology of the ligaments, tendons, and osseous structures. The anterolateral compartment of the ankle is normally a recess of the joint. However, hypertrophic synovial scar tissue caused by an injury to the lateral capsule and the components of the lateral collateral ligament can cause pain, particularly during dorsiflexion. Magnetic resonance imaging is useful for analysis of soft-tissue abnormalities involving the ankle and especially for analysis of ligamentous disruption and changes in the synovial contour of the joint. The most common pattern of anterolateral impingement is nodular—thickening of the synovium of the joint, indicating the presence of inflamed synovium and fibrous tissue. Arthroscopic ablation of the inflammatory synovial mass is the treatment of choice and is usually sufficient for pain relief. In one series, 97% of patients who had this procedure demonstrated symptomatic improvement.

Palmar Fibromatosis

1. Palmar fibromatosis, Gorham's disease, hereditary osteolysis, metastasis, any aggressive primary bone neoplasm, and soft-tissue sarcoma.

2. Yes, the tapering of the bone suggests a slow extraosseous process.

3. Fibromatosis of the palmar fascia. Plantar fibroma (Ledderhose's disease) and penile fibromatosis (Peyronie's disease).

4. No, Gorham's disease is characterized by proliferation of hemangiomatous and lymphangiomatous tissue.

Reference

Quinn SF, Erickson SJ, Dee PM, et al: MR imaging of fibromatosis: Results in 26 patients with pathologic correlation. AJR Am J Roentgenol 156:539-542, 1991.

Comments

Fibromatoses compose a group of soft-tissue lesions that may occur either as a superficial nodular mass or as a deep, infiltrative soft-tissue mass that may mimic a malignancy. Histologically, this pathologic process is characterized by fibroblastic proliferation within the muscles, the connective tissue, or both. Clinically, a majority of patients present with a small nodule beneath the skin; however, deeper lesions tend to be more insidious and may not be detected until they elicit a mass effect on the adjacent musculature or neurovascular structure. The recurrence rate for simple excision is high, ranging from 60% to 100%.

This patient has palmar fibromatosis, known as Dupuytren's contracture, which occurs when proliferative fibrous tissue involves the palmar fascia. It can be highly aggressive and can infiltrate the surrounding muscles, producing pressure erosions, cortical destruction, and bone lysis. Pathologic fractures are not uncommon. On magnetic resonance imaging, fibromatosis may have a variety of appearances, reflecting the tissue's composition and cellularity. On T1W images, lesions are isointense to slightly hyperintense in comparison with the signal intensity of muscle. Areas of low signal intensity represent dense clusters of collagen. On T2W images, a wide spectrum of signal intensity has been observed that correlates with the extent of fibrosis and cellular concentration. In comparison with the signal intensity of muscle, lesions may appear homogeneously low in signal intensity (abundant fibrous tissue), isointense to slightly hyperintense, or heterogeneously bright (extensive cellularity).

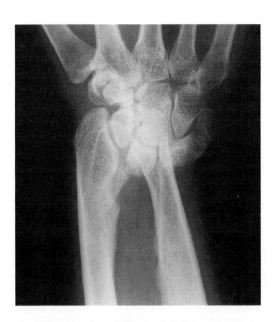 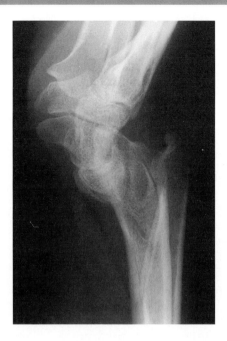

1. What is the differential diagnosis?

2. What is the essential abnormality in Turner's syndrome?

3. In Madelung's deformity, what is the principal abnormality?

4. Are patients with the idiopathic form of Madelung's deformity short in stature? Who is affected—males, females, or both?

Dyschondrosteosis

1. Dyschondrosteosis, idiopathic Madelung's deformity, and Turner's syndrome. Posttraumatic malunion and growth arrest of distal radius from epiphyseal plate trauma may mimic this deformity.

2. Only one sex chromosome (XO).

3. Bowing of the distal end of the radius while the ulna continues to grow in a straight direction.

4. No, they are normal in height. Females.

Reference

Cook PA, Yu JS, Wiand W, et al: Madelung deformity in skeletally immature patients: Morphologic assessment using radiographs, CT, and MR imaging. J Comput Assist Tomogr 20:505–511, 1996.

Comments

Dyschondrosteosis, also known as Leri-Weill syndrome, is an inherited mesomelic dwarfism characterized by bilateral Madelung's deformity of the forearms and wrists, short forearms, and short lower legs. It is transmitted as an autosomal dominant trait with a female preponderance. The range of motion at the wrists and elbows is restricted. Radiographically, the hallmark of this congenital disorder is Madelung's deformity, which is characterized by bowing of the distal radius in an ulnar and volar direction, giving rise to a relatively elongated and dorsally dislocated ulna. A pyramid-shaped carpus is a typical feature, along with abnormal tilt of the radial articular surface. Anomalous ligaments contribute to the deformity of the volar aspect of the wrist. Other findings may include curvature and shortening of the tibia and fibula. A valgus deformity of the knee joint may be present. The differential diagnosis is limited because Madelung's deformity is not typically seen in other mesomelic dwarfs. Although the deformities of the lower extremity mimic those that occur in Turner's syndrome, other distinct clinical manifestations differentiate dyschondrosteosis from Turner's syndrome.

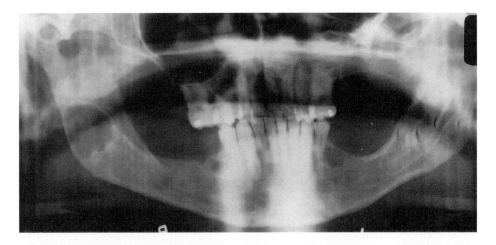

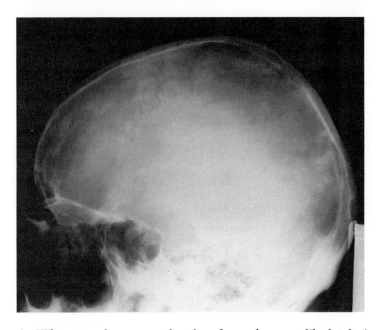

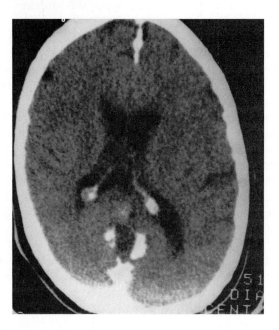

1. What neoplasm may develop from the mandibular lesions?

2. Name a few of the cutaneous manifestations of this syndrome.

3. Can the reproductive organs be affected?

4. What abnormality is common in the hands? What is the differential diagnosis?

Basal Cell Nevus (Gorlin's) Syndrome

1. Ameloblastoma.

2. Basal cell epitheliomas, milia, comedones, sebaceous cysts, and dyskeratosis.

3. Yes, ovarian and uterine fibromas in females, and hypogonadism and cryptorchidism in males.

4. A shortened metacarpal bone. Pseudohypoparathyroidism, pseudopseudohypoparathyroidism, Turner's syndrome, post infarction, post trauma, and idiopathic.

Reference

Resnick D: Soft tissues. In Diagnosis of Bone and Joint Disorders, 3rd ed. Philadelphia, WB Saunders, 1995, pp 4606–4607.

Comments

Basal cell nevus syndrome is an inherited (autosomal dominant) disorder that is characterized by multiple basal cell epitheliomas (as many as 1000), mandibular keratocysts, brachydactyly, bifid ribs, scoliosis, intracranial calcification, and numerous mesenteric cysts. The genetic defect appears to be deletions in the F 19-20 group and the marker chromosomes. Basal cell epitheliomas usually occur at about the time of puberty but may be seen in childhood. They tend to cluster in the face and trunk and may ulcerate and become locally invasive.

Radiographically, mandibular cysts vary in size from several millimeters to several centimeters and occur most commonly at the angle of the mandible. Anomalies of the spine include abnormalities in development or segmentation such as spina bifida, block vertebrae, or hemivertebrae. Spondylolisthesis and spondylolysis may also occur. Computed tomography and skull radiographs demonstrate prominent intracranial calcifications involving the falx cerebri, dura, and tentorium. Nearly 50% of patients have a shortened metacarpal bone. Intraosseous cysts have been described to have a flame-shaped appearance and may be secondary to intraosseous epithelial cysts.

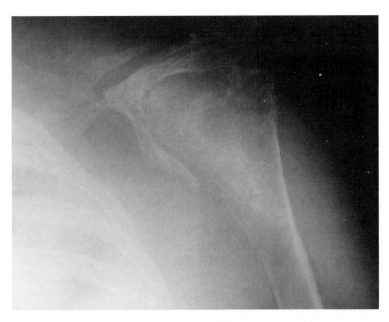 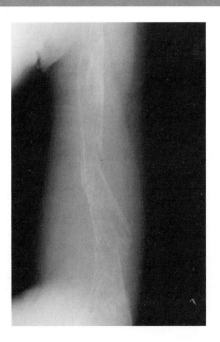

1. What is the differential diagnosis?
2. What is Gorham's syndrome? How do patients with this disease present?
3. What is characteristic of idiopathic multicentric osteolysis? And of the hereditary form?
4. What are important radiographic features of Gorham's syndrome?

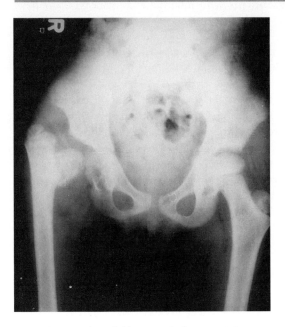

1. What is the differential diagnosis?
2. Can infection cause this deformity? How?
3. What is the essential abnormality in osteogenesis imperfecta?
4. Can patients with infantile coxa vara present with bilateral deformities? How do they present?

Gorham's Syndrome

1. Gorham's syndrome, primary osseous or soft-tissue neoplasm, metastasis, and infection.

2. Massive lysis of bone by angiomatous tissue. Variable spectrum from pain and soft-tissue swelling to insidious muscle and soft-tissue atrophy and limitation in joint motion.

3. It affects only the hand and the foot. It does not cause tapering of tubular bones.

4. Regional lysis of bone, tapering or "pointing" of the remaining bone (particularly tubular bone), and atrophy of soft tissue.

Reference

Chung C, Yu JS, Resnick D, et al: Gorham syndrome of the thorax and cervical spine: CT and MRI findings. Skeletal Radiol 26:55–59, 1997.

Comments

The main observation in this case is regional osteolysis about the shoulder joint. This finding is characteristic of Gorham's syndrome, which is also known as massive osteolysis and vanishing bone disease. Definitive diagnosis is based on histopathology. No age is spared; the age range of patients at presentation has been from 1 year to 75 years. Nearly two thirds of patients affected have been males, and more than 50% have a prior history of trauma to the involved area. The skeletal distribution has favored the shoulder girdle (26%) and the mandible (15%), although any bone may be affected. The process is primarily monocentric and is considered benign, but its progressive nature and resistance to treatment mimic a neoplasm. Complications can be severe and may result in death.

Theories that have been proposed to explain its etiology include traumatic hyperemia, mechanical causes, changes in blood pH, hyperoxia, unrestricted growth of granulation tissue, and endothelial cell–mediated resorption of the bone matrix. Typically, as bone lysis occurs, the demineralized area is replaced by a vascular fibrous stroma characterized by the presence of numerous blood vessels. Radiographically, the disease begins with patchy osteoporosis followed by progressive soft-tissue atrophy and fracture, fragmentation, and disappearance of bone. The process then extends to contiguous bones, resulting in regional destruction, which is characteristic of this disease.

Infantile Coxa Vara

1. Infantile coxa vara, proximal femoral focal deficiency, osteogenesis imperfecta, renal osteodystrophy, rickets, and fibrous dysplasia.

2. Yes, arrested growth when the epiphyseal plate is destroyed.

3. Fragile bones predisposed to fracture either from abnormal maturation of collagen or from unstable cross-linking of collagen.

4. Yes, both hip joints are affected in one third of cases. "Duck waddle" gait.

Reference

Pavlov H, Goldman AB, Freiberger RH: Infantile coxa vara. Radiology 135:631–640, 1980.

Comments

The age of this patient (skeletally immature) and the classic deformity of the proximal femur are virtually pathognomonic of infantile coxa vara, an unusual localized dysplasia. The deformity is characterized by a diminished femoral neck angle (the angle subtended by the long axis of the femoral neck and shaft). This angle is about 150 degrees at birth and decreases to a range of 120 to 130 degrees in the normal adult. In patients with this deformity, the angle measures less than 120 degrees. Patients with infantile coxa vara typically have a severe varus deformity associated with an irregularly widened growth plate and thickening of the medial cortex of the femoral neck bridging the head to the shaft. The acetabulum is flattened, and the greater trochanter is relatively enlarged. A characteristic triangular osseous fragment at the medial inferior corner of the metaphysis is a frequent finding. In this condition, patients present early in life with a gait abnormality and restricted range of motion. The cause is unknown, but etiologies that have been suggested include osteochondrosis, pathologic ossification of the femoral neck, interrupted vascular supply, and trauma.

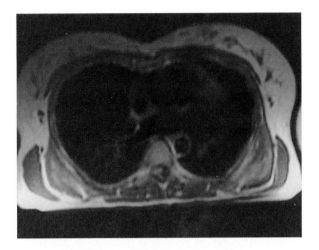
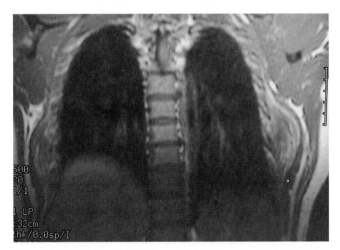

1. What is the most likely diagnosis?

2. What is most characteristic about this tumor?

3. Is computed tomography (CT) or magnetic resonance imaging (MRI) the preferred technique for diagnosing this lesion?

4. Would you biopsy this lesion?

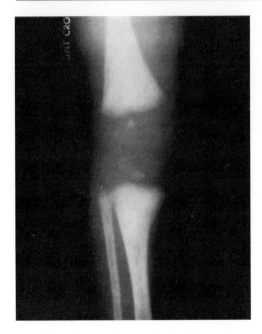
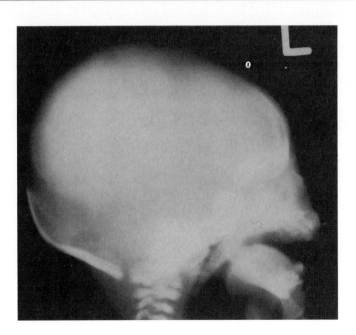

1. What is the differential diagnosis?

2. Is the abnormality in the metaphysis permanent?

3. Which congenital infection can be further complicated by the development of a progressive, subacute panencephalitis in the second decade of life?

4. What are osseous findings of congenital syphilis?

C A S E 1 7 9

Elastofibroma Dorsi

1. Elastofibroma dorsi.

2. Its location about the shoulder and its striated MRI appearance.

3. MRI. CT lacks sufficient soft-tissue contrast to define the margins of the tumor from the adjacent musculature, but it is excellent for detecting invasion of the osseous structures. On MRI, linear or curvilinear regions of alternating high and intermediate signal intensity on T1W images reflect the histologic composition of fat and fibrous tissue.

4. If the patient is middle-aged and there are no symptoms associated with the mass, I would just watch it.

Reference

Yu JS, Weis LD, Vaughan LM, Resnick D: MRI of elastofibroma dorsi. J Comput Assist Tomogr 19:601-603, 1995.

Comments

Elastofibroma dorsi is a rare, benign, fibroproliferative tumor of unknown pathogenesis. In 85% of cases, elastofibromas arise beneath the rhomboid major and latissimus dorsi muscles, subjacent to the inferior angle of the scapula. Other reported sites of involvement include the soft tissues about the ischial tuberosity, infraolecranon area, deltoid muscle, axilla, intraspinal space, orbit, foot, stomach, greater trochanter, greater omentum, and chest wall. This slow-growing tumor is usually a unilateral process, although bilateral involvement or involvement of multiple sites is not infrequent. Most patients are asymptomatic, but when symptoms are present, stiffness and pain with motion are common complaints. On gross pathology, an elastofibroma is a nonencapsulated tumor characterized by varying quantities of fat and fibrous tissue. Microscopically, an elastofibroma is characterized by the presence of numerous branched and unbranched eosinophilic fibers that acquire an irregularly globular or beadlike appearance when exposed to an elastin stain, a feature that is useful in distinguishing elastofibromas from other fibrous pseudotumors or neoplasms. The background tumor matrix is composed of variable quantities of fibrous connective tissue intermingled with mature adipose tissue; these are tissues that are amenable to MRI imaging. Most lesions are treated conservatively.

C A S E 1 8 0

Congenital Rubella

1. Congenital rubella, cytomegalic inclusion disease, congenital syphilis, congenital herpes simplex, occasionally vaccinial osteomyelitis, and occasionally neonatal rickets.

2. No, it resolves when the child recovers from the infection.

3. Patients with congenital rubella may develop ataxia, seizure, spasticity, and deterioration of intellectual function.

4. Osteochondritis at the epiphyseal-metaphyseal junction with irregular metaphyseal erosions, diaphyseal osteomyelitis-periostitis, and reparative periostitis.

References

Chapman S: Celery-stick long bones. Br J Hosp Med 45:380-382, 1991.

Reef SE: Rubella and congenital rubella syndrome. Bull World Health Organ 76:156-157, 1998.

Comments

Rubella, or German measles, is a benign infectious condition in the adult, but infection during the first trimester of pregnancy may have significant consequences in the development of the fetal skeleton and other cell lines. Congenital rubella is caused by transplacental transmission of the togavirus to the fetus in the presence of active maternal infection. The infection may lead to growth retardation, hepatosplenomegaly, and structural malformations of the cardiovascular (patent ductus arteriosus, ventricular septal defect, pulmonic stenosis), ocular (corneal clouding, chorioretinitis, microphthalmia, cataract), and central nervous (mental retardation, microcephaly, deafness) systems. The radiographic findings are most pronounced in the metaphyseal portions of the femur and tibia. The lesions are characterized by linear lucent areas alternating with linear bands of increased density, producing a striated pattern that is referred to as a "celery stalk" appearance. Radiolucent metaphyseal bands are also evident in this patient. (In patients with rickets, this finding is associated with widening of the growth plate.) There is conspicuous absence of periostitis, a finding that helps to exclude osteomyelitis. The absence of intracranial calcifications in the lateral skull radiograph decreases the likelihood of cytomegalic inclusion disease.

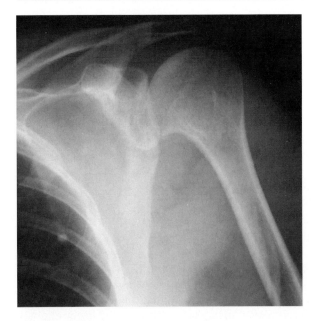

1. What observation did you make?
2. Might this abnormality be the result of prior trauma?
3. Is this commonly a unilateral or a bilateral process?
4. Is this deformity associated with any other skeletal anomaly?

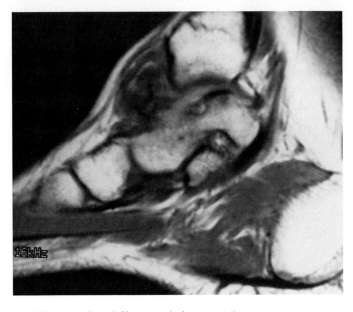 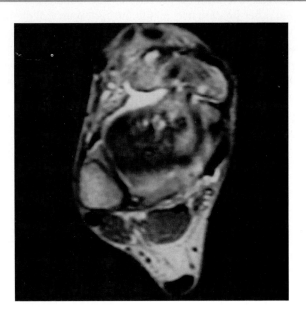

1. What is the differential diagnosis?
2. Can this lesion undergo malignant transformation?
3. How does ossification occur?
4. Is there an association between an intra-articular osteochondroma and Hoffa's disease?

Glenoid Hypoplasia

1. Hypoplasia of the glenoid neck (dentate anomaly).

2. Only if the glenoid ossification center was previously injured from a fracture.

3. Bilateral.

4. Hypoplasia of the humeral head and neck, varus deformity of the proximal portion of the humerus, and enlargement and bowing of the acromion and the clavicle.

Reference

Trout TE, Resnick D: Glenoid hypoplasia and its relationship to instability. Skeletal Radiol 25:37–40, 1996.

Comments

This "aunt Minnie" is uncommon and affects men and women with equal frequency. There often is a familial tendency, suggesting a hereditary trait. This condition represents anomalous development of the scapula with hypoplasia or dysplasia of the glenoid neck. The glenoid fossa develops in a broad, irregular fashion, resulting in a widened inferior glenohumeral joint, and the articular surface becomes notched. Patients present with shoulder pain and limited range of motion, and instability is more common than was previously suspected. The radiographic findings are classic and diagnostic. Only one other process may mimic the appearance of glenoid hypoplasia. An injury to the brachial plexus occurring at birth may produce radiographic abnormalities that are similar to this anomaly, but these patients also have upper extremity paralysis, with atrophic musculature that provides a differentiating finding.

Intra-articular Osteochondroma

1. Intra-articular osteochondroma, intra-articular body, osteochondromatosis, and Trevor's disease.

2. No.

3. Either by enchondral ossification or by periosteal new bone formation.

4. Some believe that this lesion represents an end stage of Hoffa's disease.

Reference

Reith JD, Bauer TW, Joyce MJ: Paraarticular osteochondroma of the knee: Report of 2 cases and review of the literature. Clin Orthop 334:225–232, 1997.

Comments

An intra-articular osteochondroma is an uncommon entity. Some have hypothesized that this lesion is the result of extrasynovial metaplasia, although the exact etiology of this lesion remains unknown. The most common location of an intra-articular osteochondroma is the knee within the infrapatellar fat pad of Hoffa. Clinically, most patients present with a nontender mass, persistent swelling, or diminished range of motion. A history of remote trauma is elicited in only a small number of patients. The mass tends to be fixed in location and firm. Intra-articular osteochondromas have a variety of radiographic and magnetic resonance imaging (MRI) appearances. Some lesions have the characteristic appearance of an extra-articular osteochondroma. In other lesions, the MRI manifestation is that of an intra-articular mass with or without a fibrous attachment to the synovium or the capsule of the joint. On T1W images, the signal intensity of the mass is isointense to muscle, but there may be punctate areas of low signal intensity scattered throughout the center of the osteochondroma representing calcification, or there may be a peripheral rim of low signal intensity representing mature periosteum. The appearance on T2W images is quite variable, and the lesion may be either low or high in signal intensity. Enhancement is also highly variable.

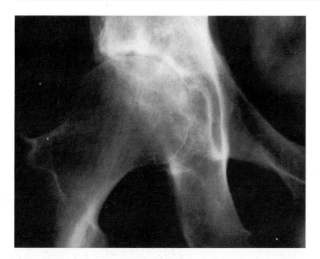
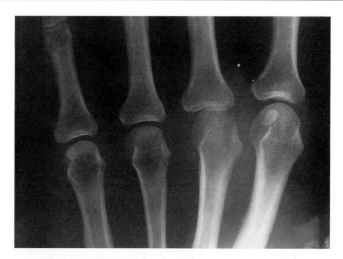

1. Synovial fluid aspiration from the hip shows a white blood cell (WBC) count of 2000 to 10,000 cells per cubic millimeter and consists mostly of granulocytes. What is the diagnosis in this patient, who had presented with a new erythematous skin lesion?

2. What is Lyme disease, and what are its characteristic features?

3. How often does arthritis develop with Lyme disease?

4. What joints are typically involved in Lyme disease?

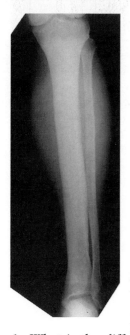
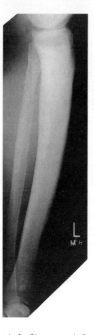

1. What is the differential diagnosis?

2. Of the sclerosing bone conditions, which present in middle-aged adults?

3. Histologically, what is seen in areas of sclerosis in patients with Erdheim-Chester disease?

4. What pediatric disease do the pathologic findings of Erdheim-Chester disease resemble?

C A S E 1 8 3

Lyme Disease

1. Lyme arthropathy.

2. An expanding erythematous skin lesion, arthritis, neurologic abnormalities (Bell's palsy, meningitis), and cardiac conduction abnormalities.

3. Fifty percent of patients develop arthritis.

4. By order of decreasing frequency—knee, shoulder, elbow, temporomandibular joint, ankle, wrist, hip, and small joints of the hand and foot.

Reference

Eustace SJ, Lan HH, Dorfman D: Lyme arthropathy. Radiol Clin North Am 34:454–455, 1996.

Comments

Lyme disease is an infectious condition caused by the spirochete *Borrelia burgdorferi.* Although both children and adults may be infected, there is a tendency for the disease to affect children and young adults during the summer and fall, because these age groups are more likely to spend time outdoors in wooded areas, where they may encounter the tick *Ixodes dammini.* The disease begins with a small papule in the area of the tick bite, usually on the trunk. This papule becomes an expanding, erythematous, annular lesion called erythema chronicum migrans, which may reach a diameter of 50 cm. About 75% of patients have this characteristic skin lesion. Fever, chills, headache, and malaise often accompany the skin lesion. Splenomegaly and cardiac conduction abnormalities may also occur in the acute phase of the disease. An acute, monoarticular or oligoarticular, inflammatory arthropathy develops about 2 to 6 months after the skin lesion. It is typically of short duration (1 week) but tends to recur and may have a migratory nature. Significant joint damage does not occur in a majority of patients, but some patients develop a chronic, synovial inflammatory process with significant destruction of the cartilage and subchondral bone by pannus. The differential diagnosis is based on clinical and radiographic findings and includes juvenile chronic arthritis, Reiter's syndrome, rheumatic fever, and granulomatous infections.

C A S E 1 8 4

Erdheim-Chester Disease

1. Erdheim-Chester disease, Engelmann's disease, Ribbing's disease, fluorosis, hyperphosphatasemia, van Buchem's syndrome, osteopetrosis, myelosclerosis, and mastocytosis.

2. Erdheim-Chester disease, myelosclerosis, and—occasionally—fluorosis and van Buchem's syndrome.

3. Cells rich in cholesterol, interspersed with lymphocytes and plasma cells within the cortex, and connective tissue cells, intermixed with foam cells within the spongiosa.

4. Hand-Schüller-Christian disease.

References

Bancroft LW, Berquist TH: Erdheim-Chester disease: Radiographic findings in five patients. Skeletal Radiol 27:127–132, 1998.

Franzius C, Sciuk J, Bremer C, et al: Determination of extent and activity with radionuclide imaging in Erdheim-Chester disease. Clin Nucl Med 24:252–255, 1999.

Comments

Erdheim-Chester disease is a histiocytic condition of unknown etiology that affects middle-aged men and women. The disease is characterized by the deposition of cholesterol-laden foam cells in the bone marrow, heart, lungs, kidneys, and xanthomatous patches in the eyelids. The most distinctive feature of this rare disease is osteosclerosis of the long bones of the appendicular skeleton. Involvement of the axial skeleton is uncommon. Radiographically, a symmetrical increase in bone density occurs either diffusely or in a patchy distribution, with associated coarsening of the trabeculation, sclerosis of the medullary cavity, and cortical thickening in the diaphysis and metaphysis of the bones. Involvement of the epiphysis is uncommon. Bone scintigraphy demonstrates activity in these sclerotic areas. Magnetic resonance imaging also demonstrates the pathologic areas well. On T1W images, the abnormal bone demonstrates hypointense signal intensity, which becomes heterogeneously hyperintense and hypointense on T2W images. The diagnosis requires histologic confirmation.

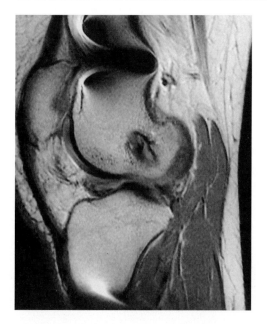 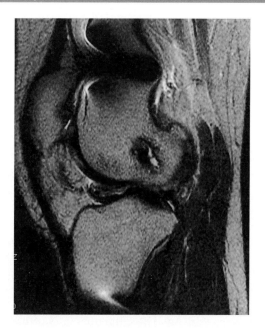

1. What kind of surgery did this patient have?
2. What complication did he develop? What is its arthroscopic appearance?
3. What causes this abnormality?
4. How does roof impingement occur, and does it become apparent with full flexion or with extension?

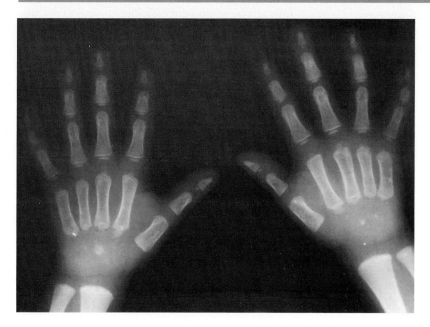

1. What is your diagnosis? On what observation did you base your conclusion?
2. List some of the findings you may observe in the skull.
3. What complication can affect the hip joints?
4. What conditions can cause fragmentation (or stippling) of the epiphyses?

Localized Anterior Arthrofibrosis (Cyclops Lesion)

1. Anterior cruciate ligament (ACL) reconstruction.

2. Localized anterior arthrofibrosis, or a cyclops lesion. A headlike nodule with reddish-blue discoloration that resembles the eye of the cyclops.

3. Either debris raised by drilling the tibial tunnel or injury to the exposed fibers of an ACL graft by roof impingement.

4. The tibial tunnel is placed too far anterior on the tibia, causing effacement and constriction of an ACL graft during the last 5 to 10 degrees of knee extension.

Reference

Recht MP, Piraino DW, Applegate G, et al: Complications after anterior cruciate ligament reconstruction: Radiographic and MR findings. AJR Am J Roentgenol 167:705–710, 1996.

Comments

The key observation in this patient is a nodular mass in the anterior joint recess adjacent to the ACL graft. On the proton density images, the mass demonstrates isointense signal intensity to muscle. On the corresponding T2W image, it shows heterogeneous signal intensity. Localized anterior arthrofibrosis, otherwise known as a cyclops lesion because of its appearance on arthroscopy, represents a focal, reactive, fibrous nodule that is often attached to the ACL graft. It is an important cause of diminished range of motion and occasionally of joint locking in postoperative patients. The greater frequency of ACL reconstructions has increased the need to be informed about the imaging features of this procedure in both normal and pathologic situations.

Hypothyroidism

1. Hypothyroidism (juvenile myxedema). Markedly delayed skeletal maturation, particularly involving the carpus.

2. Brachycephaly, enlargement of the sella turcica, wormian bones, underdeveloped sinuses, prognathism, and delayed dental development.

3. Slipped capital femoral epiphysis.

4. Hypothyroidism, multiple epiphyseal dysplasia, osteonecrosis, chondrodysplasia punctata, and chondrodystrophia calcificans congenita.

Reference

Desai MP, Joshi NC: Roentgenologic changes in hypothyroidism (a study of 40 cases). Indian Pediatr 9:201–207, 1972.

Comments

Hypothyroidism is caused by a variety of structural or functional abnormalities that result in insufficient synthesis of thyroid hormone. The congenital form produces developmental abnormalities from birth and is termed *cretinism*. When it is acquired in youth, the disease is characterized by the accumulation of hydrophilic mucopolysaccharides in the dermis and is termed *juvenile myxedema*. Manifestations of cretinism (jaundice, hoarse cry, somnolence, failure to thrive) are usually evident within the first few months of life. In children, mental retardation and characteristic physical features (enlarged tongue, broad nose, widely set eyes, sparse hair, dry skin, protuberant abdomen, short stature) become apparent.

The key to the diagnosis in this case is markedly delayed skeletal maturation. Only two carpal bones have barely ossified in each wrist, and the epiphyses of the distal radius and ulna have not yet begun to ossify. The development of the fingers and the thumb, however, indicate that this patient is much older (he is 6 years old). Retardation of skeletal development is a hallmark of both congenital and juvenile forms of hypothyroidism. Absence of the distal femoral and proximal tibial epiphyses is an important observation in patients with cretinism. As the patient matures, abnormal development of the bone is characterized by fragmentation of the ossification centers (epiphyseal dysgenesis).

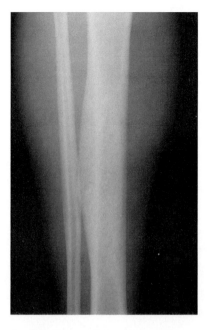
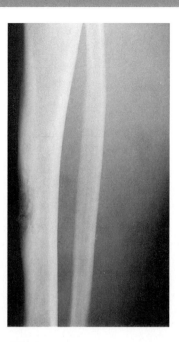

1. What conditions would you consider?

2. Under what conditions can the bone become secondarily infected from a soft-tissue focus?

3. How does a cortical abscess develop, and what is its natural course if untreated?

4. Is periostitis from an infection more pronounced in children or in adults?

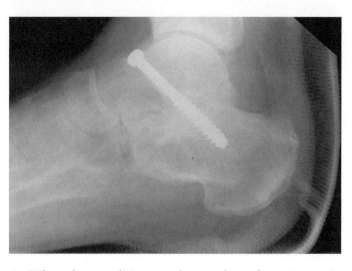
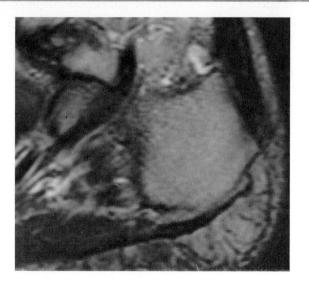

1. What abnormalities are depicted on these images?

2. Define a "pump bump." List the differential diagnosis of a pump bump.

3. Does the retrocalcaneal bursa contain a synovial lining?

4. What general observations help differentiate tears of the Achilles' tendon from tendinosis?

Cortical Abscess

1. Chronic sclerosing osteomyelitis, cortical abscess, and—less likely—osteoid osteoma and stress-induced periostitis.

2. Trauma, animal or human bites, puncture wounds, irradiation, and burns.

3. An adjacent soft-tissue infection invades the periosteum (periostitis), which causes formation of a subperiosteal abscess (cortical erosion) that penetrates the haversian and Volkmann's canals (cortical abscess) and finally perforates the marrow (lysis and osteomyelitis).

4. In children, because the periosteal attachment is less rigid.

References

Kozlowski K, Hochberger O: Rare forms of chronic osteomyelitis (multifocal recurrent periostitis and chronic symmetric osteomyelitis—report of 3 cases). Australas Radiol 28:152-155, 1984.

Nortje CJ, Wood RE, Grotepass F: Periostitis ossificans versus Garre's osteomyelitis. Oral Surg Oral Med Oral Pathol 66:249-260, 1988.

Comments

When osteomyelitis develops from a contiguous source of infection, the radiographic presentation depends on the length of time that the adjacent tissue has been infected, on the part of the bone that becomes infected, on the virulence of the organism, and on the age of the patient. This case demonstrates an uncommon presentation of chronic osteomyelitis caused by a contiguous source of infection. Chronic sclerosing osteomyelitis is more common in the mandible. This patient developed a cortical abscess from a penetrating injury. The main observations included prominent periosteal thickening, lysis of the cortex at the site of the abscess, formation of a sequestrum, and a sinus tract that allowed communication between the cortical abscess and the adjacent soft tissue. At first glance, the development of considerable periosteal new bone mimics an osteoid osteoma, but the absence of a nidus and the distinctly different clinical presentation separate these entities. The length of bone involved and the atypical location affected also render the diagnosis of a stress fracture unlikely. A cortical metastasis is unusual and does not elicit periosteal reactive changes.

Haglund's Disease

1. Achilles' tendinosis and retrocalcaneal bursitis caused by a prominent calcaneal bursal projection (Haglund's disease).

2. A soft-tissue or bony prominence in the back of the heel. Haglund's deformity, seronegative inflammatory arthropathies such as Reiter's syndrome, retrocalcaneal bursitis, superficial Achilles' bursitis, and Achilles' tendon abnormalities (tear, tendinosis, ossification).

3. Yes.

4. Most tears occur 2 to 6 cm above the calcaneal insertion, whereas tendinosis tends to occur more distally at the enthesis.

Reference

Yu JS, Vitellas KM: The calcaneus: Applications of magnetic resonance imaging. Foot Ankle Int 17:771-780, 1996.

Comments

Haglund's disease is caused by an abnormal prominence of the posterior superior border (bursal projection) of the calcaneus. Constant rubbing of the back of a shoe irritates this area of the foot, causing posterior heel pain. This condition is often associated with retrocalcaneal bursitis and Achilles' tendinosis. There are two techniques for determining an abnormal bursal projection. In the posterior calcaneal angle technique, a Haglund's deformity is present when the angle subtended by a baseline tangent (line drawn from the inferior surface of the anterior tubercle to the medial tubercle) and a posterior tangent (the line drawn from the posterior surface of the posterior tubercle to the bursal projection) exceeds 75 degrees. In the parallel pitch line technique, a line parallel to the baseline tangent drawn from the posterior lip of the apex of the posterior calcaneal facet defines the superior limit of the bursal projection. Any portion of the calcaneus that extends above the parallel pitch line is considered pathologic and indicative of Haglund's deformity.

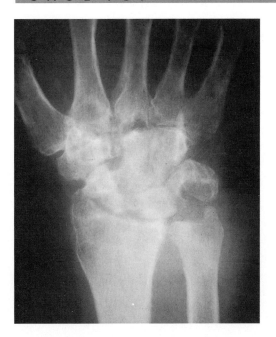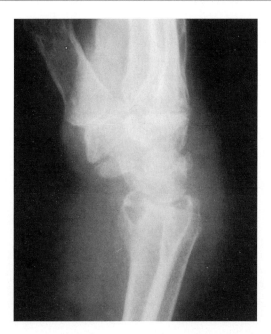

1. What are the significant findings?
2. What is a serious complication of tuberculous spondylitis? List the processes that lead to this complication.
3. What is a tubercle?
4. How would you make a definitive diagnosis of tuberculous arthritis?

Tuberculous Arthritis

1. The Phemister triad (juxta-articular osteoporosis, marginal erosions, and relative preservation of the joint spaces) and marked soft-tissue swelling.

2. Spinal cord compression. Abscesses, granulation tissue or bone fragments, arachnoiditis, endarteritis-induced ischemia, and intramedullary granulomas.

3. A well-demarcated mass containing bacilli formed by multinucleated giant cells surrounded by lymphocytes and epithelioid cells.

4. A synovial biopsy.

References

Meltzer RM, Deehl LJ, Karlin JM, et al: Tuberculous arthritis: A case study and review of the literature. J Foot Surg 24:30–39, 1985.

Suh JS, Lee JD, Cho JH, et al: MR imaging of tuberculous arthritis: Clinical and experimental studies. J Magn Reson Imaging 6:185–189, 1996.

Comments

Skeletal tuberculosis is an uncommon but important cause of osteomyelitis in the immunocompromised host. Infection occurs by a hematogenous route arising from a primary infection in the lung or urogenital focus. Infections caused by a *Mycobacterium* agent tend to have a slower course and less pronounced host reaction than do those caused by pyogenic infections. Common complaints include pain, swelling, weakness, muscle atrophy, and a draining sinus. The disease is characterized by the formation of tubercles with central caseating necrosis. Tuberculous osteomyelitis can remain localized to the bone or may spread to adjacent joints. In children, transphyseal spread of infection favors a granulomatous, not a bacterial, etiology.

This case is difficult, and the only method to definitively confirm this diagnosis is a synovial biopsy. Periarticular osteoporosis and joint effusion indicate the presence of synovial inflammation. As the inflamed synovial tissue spreads, erosions through the cartilage into the subchondral bone produce marginal erosions demarcated by a rim of sclerosis. Relative preservation of the joint space despite marked erosive changes is an important observation. On magnetic resonance imaging, intermediate signal intensity tissue in areas of erosion on T2W images is strongly suggestive of tuberculosis. Remember that rheumatoid arthritis and idiopathic chondrolysis cause early loss of joint space. In gout, osteopenia is not a predominant finding.

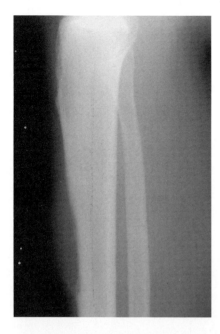
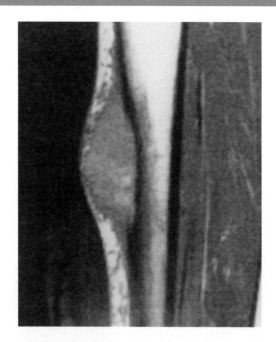
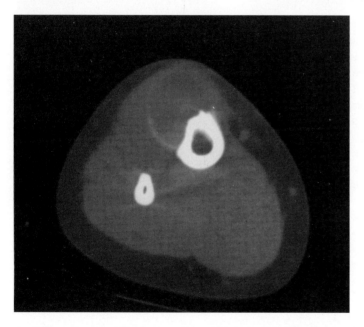

1. What do you observe, and what lesions would you consider?

2. List some observations that do not support a diagnosis of periosteal osteosarcoma.

3. What feature favors an osteoblastoma over a periosteal chondroma?

4. The radiographic features of a malignant osteoblastoma resemble what other tumors?

Benign Subperiosteal Osteoblastoma

1. Saucerization of the bone; consider periosteal chondroma, periosteal chondrosarcoma, periosteal desmoid, benign osteoblastoma, and neurofibroma.

2. The absence of radiating osseous spicules that extends into the soft tissues and the smoothness of the cortical saucerization.

3. The size of the lesion. Periosteal chondroma seldom exceeds 4 cm.

4. Osteosarcoma and Ewing's sarcoma.

Reference

Goldman RL: The periosteal counterpart of benign osteoblastoma. Am J Clin Pathol 56:73–78, 1971.

Comments

A benign osteoblastoma is an uncommon neoplasm characterized by the presence of osteoblasts and giant cells in vascular connective tissue. It affects young people (younger than 30 years) and has a twofold predilection for men. Pain is a common complaint, but relief with salicylates is an inconstant finding. The most common location for this tumor is the spine, although long tubular bones are involved in one third of cases. When benign osteoblastoma involves a long bone, 75% of lesions are located in the diaphysis, and the remainder involve the metaphysis. The radiographic features of this lesion depend on its location, which can be cortical, medullary, or subperiosteal. When this lesion is in the bone, it tends to be well marginated, to have a narrow zone of transition, and to be demarcated by a rim of sclerosis. The lesion can be expansile and demonstrate areas of calcification or ossification. Periostitis may be exuberant, particularly at the margin of the mass, producing fusiform thickening of the cortex. The findings in this case are not very specific, and it is not possible to render a precise diagnosis. But the important observation that you should have made is the large area of saucerization. The presence of this area increases the likelihood of an osteoblastoma, and because this lesion has a potential for malignant transformation, a biopsy should be performed next for a pathologic diagnosis.

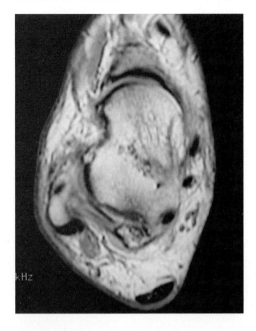 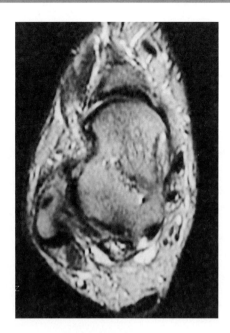

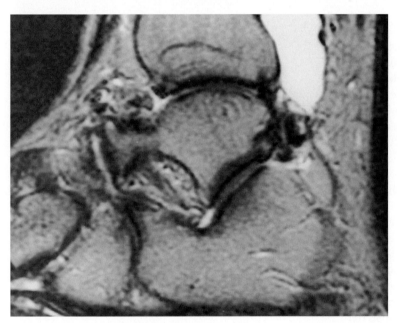

1. What is the most likely diagnosis? Why is the flexor hallucis longus tendon involved?

2. What is a Shepherd's fracture?

3. What attaches to the os trigonum?

4. Name two mechanisms of injury that can fracture the trigonal process.

Os Trigonum Syndrome

1. Os trigonum syndrome with tenosynovitis of the flexor hallucis longus tendon. Location—the flexor hallucis longus tendon sits medial to the ossicle in the sulcus between the medial tubercle and the larger lateral tubercle of the posterior talus.

2. A fracture of the lateral talar tubercle.

3. Posterior talofibular and posterior talocalcaneal ligaments.

4. Forced plantar flexion of the foot causes talar compression between the tibia and the calcaneus, and forced dorsiflexion of the ankle can avulse the process through its attachment to the posterior talofibular ligament.

Reference

Karasick D, Schweitzer ME: The os trigonum syndrome: Imaging features. AJR Am J Roentogenol 166:125–129, 1996.

Comments

The os trigonum is analogous to a secondary ossification center, having been formed within a cartilaginous extension from the posterior portion of the talus. It becomes mineralized between the ages of 7 and 13 years and fuses with the talus within a year of mineralization, forming the trigonal process of the talus. It remains a separate ossicle in about 7% to 15% of people, with a cartilaginous synchondrosis existing between the os and the talus.

The os trigonum syndrome is a condition characterized by chronic or recurrent pain with stiffness, tenderness, and soft-tissue swelling in the posterior ankle. It commonly affects people who perform activities that subject the ankle to extreme plantar flexion (e.g., ballet). Pain is produced by disruption of the cartilaginous synchondrosis between the os trigonum and the lateral talar tubercle, which can then produce compression of the adjacent synovial and capsular tissues against the posterior tibia. With repeated entrapment, the soft tissue becomes chronically inflamed and fibrosed, particularly the tendon of the flexor hallucis longus muscle. Contributing etiologic factors include fracture of the trigonal process, posterior tibiotalar impingement by a bone block, and intra-articular loose bodies. On magnetic resonance imaging, degenerative changes, fluid, or both may be evident at the synchondrosis, as well as bone marrow edema in the os trigonum (as in this patient). A markedly distended flexor hallucis longus tendon sheath suggests entrapment.

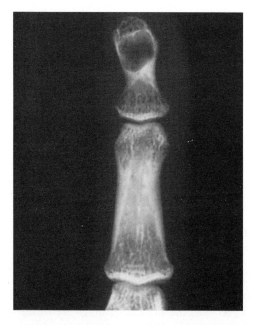

1. What conditions would you consider?
2. Describe the pathologic findings of an epidermoid cyst.
3. After this radiographic series, this patient's symptoms increased dramatically. What could have happened?
4. Why can a glomus tumor occur in the terminal phalanx?

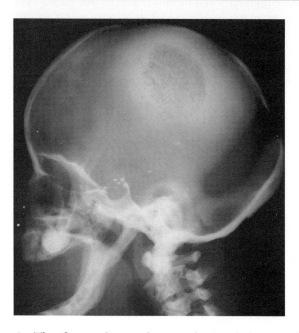 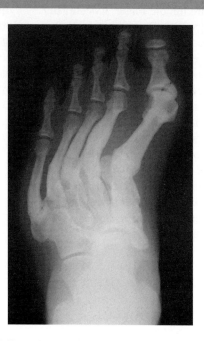

1. The first radiograph was obtained during childhood and the second during adulthood. What is your diagnosis?
2. List the conditions that cause diffuse osteosclerosis and osteolysis.
3. What abnormalities may occur in the spine of patients with this disorder?
4. What is happening in the parietal bones of this patient?

Epidermoid Inclusion Cyst

1. Epidermoid inclusion cyst, giant cell tumor, reparative granuloma, enchondroma, glomus tumor, and—rarely—metastasis.

2. A cavity filled with white, keratinous debris that is lined by stratified squamous epithelium and a thick layer of fibrous tissue.

3. Pathologic fracture or cyst rupture. Rupture of an epidermoid cyst into the connective tissue stroma elicits an intense inflammatory reaction to the released keratin.

4. Neuromyoarterial masses (glomus) are located in the fingertips, functioning as temperature regulators.

Reference

Palmieri TJ: Common tumors of the hand. Orthop Rev 16:367–378, 1987.

Comments

Epidermoid cysts are uncommon bone lesions, hypothesized to occur as a result of intraosseous implantation of ectodermal tissue from either penetrating or blunt trauma. They occur in the skull and the phalanges of the hand in most cases. The frontal and parietal bones are the most frequent sites of involvement in the skull, and the terminal phalanx is the preferred site in the hand, particularly that of the middle finger. Cysts in the hand rarely exceed 2 cm in size. They can cause mild expansion of the bone and cortical thinning, which can lead to a fracture. A thin rim of sclerosis reflects the chronicity of this lesion. Cysts in the skull can involve either or both tables and frequently can reach sizes up to 5 cm in diameter. In this case, we can provide only a differential diagnosis because lesions that produce a well-defined lytic process surrounded by sclerosis in the terminal phalanx do not have many differentiating qualities. There are several rules that may be helpful, however. Enchondroma is rare in this location. Metastases usually do not have a sclerotic rim. Glomus tumor is frequently eccentrically located or entirely extraosseous.

Pyknodysostosis

1. Pyknodysostosis.

2. Hyperparathyroidism and pyknodysostosis.

3. Abnormal segmentation and spondylolisthesis.

4. Hematopoietic activity.

Reference

Kawahara K, Nishikiori M, Imai K, et al: Radiographic observations of pyknodysostosis. Report of a case. Oral Surg Oral Med Oral Pathol 44:476–482, 1977.

Comments

Two observations are important in this case. One is osteosclerosis, which is present in the bones of the foot, and the second is abnormal development of the skull. There is prominent hypoplasia of the mandible and the facial bones and widening of the sutures and the fontanelles. In the foot, the notable findings are numerous transverse fractures in bones of the foot and acroosteolysis.

Pyknodysostosis is a rare hereditary syndrome (autosomal recessive) consisting of increased bone density, short stature, frontal and occipital bosselation, hypoplasia of the mandible, dysplasia of the skull bones, and hypoplasia-aplasia (or acro-osteolysis) of the terminal phalanges. An increased tendency toward developing multiple transverse fractures is characteristic of this condition. Although generalized osteosclerosis is a feature of pyknodysostosis, a bone-in-bone appearance does not occur, and metaphyseal modeling, if present, is mild, distinguishing this condition from osteopetrosis. Wormian bones are common in the lambdoid sutures. Mentation is normal in these patients.

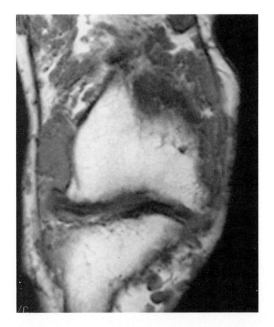
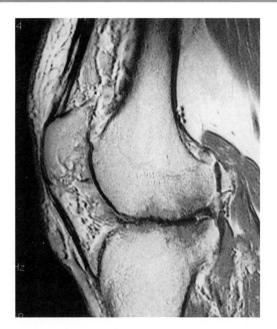
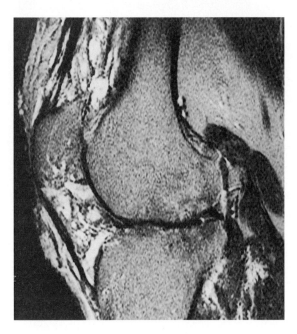

1. What is your differential diagnosis?

2. What is the difference between capillary and cavernous hemangiomas?

3. What causes a phlebolith in a hemangioma?

4. Describe Klippel-Trénaunay-Weber syndrome.

Synovial Hemangioma

1. Synovial hemangioma, pigmented villonodular synovitis, hemophilia.

2. Capillary hemangiomas are composed of disorganized capillaries with sparse fibrous stroma, and cavernous hemangiomas are composed of large, dilated, blood-filled spaces lined by flat endothelia.

3. Dystrophic calcification in organized thrombi.

4. Varicose veins, soft-tissue and osseous hypertrophy, and cutaneous hemangiomas.

Reference

Greenspan A, Azouz EM, Matthews J 2nd, Decarie JC: Synovial hemangioma: Imaging features in eight histologically proven cases, review of the literature, and differential diagnosis. Skeletal Radiol 24:583–590, 1995.

Comments

Synovial hemangiomas are uncommon, intra-articular, vascular tumors. These lesions tend to occur in adolescent or young women, causing pain, swelling, and a diminished range of motion. There are two pathologic types. One type presents as a pedunculated synovial mass and with symptoms that mimic a meniscal tear (locking and pain). The other pattern is more diffuse and is associated with synovial proliferation. The latter type may present with intermittent pain, hemarthrosis, and—occasionally—increased limb length. Associated cutaneous and soft-tissue hemangiomas are commonly seen with the diffuse form.

The radiographic features of a synovial hemangioma are similar to those of hemophilia. Joint space narrowing secondary to cartilage destruction, epiphyseal overgrowth, and synovial proliferation are common findings. In the past, the diagnosis was suggested when a villonodular pattern was depicted on arthrography. Conventional radiographs depict phleboliths or bony erosions in 50% of cases. Angiography shows fine-caliber, smooth-walled vessels with contrast pooling in dilated vascular spaces. Today, magnetic resonance imaging is preferred because it is capable of showing the extent of the lesion, the deposition of hemosiderin, and the severity of joint destruction. Fluid-fluid levels are occasional findings in cavernous-type lesions.

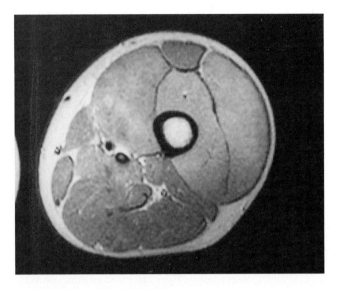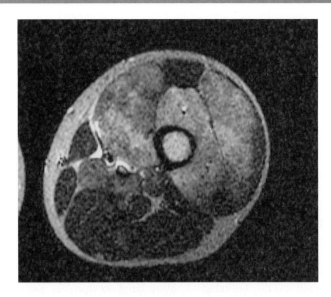

1. What are the findings?

2. What is the likely diagnosis in this weightlifter? How do you suppose this injury came about?

3. Are the magnetic resonance imaging findings permanent?

4. Over the next few days, what symptoms will this patient experience?

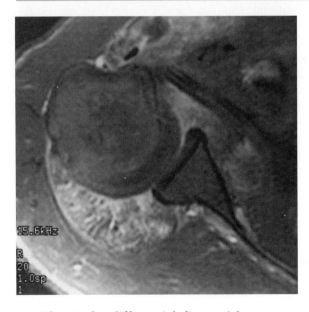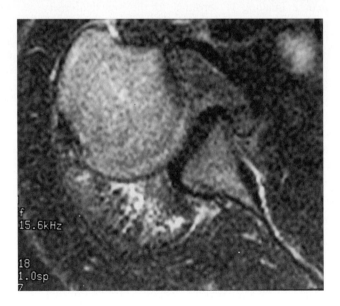

1. What is the differential diagnosis?

2. Why is pigmented villonodular synovitis an unlikely diagnosis?

3. What is the characteristic T2W appearance of the cartilaginous components in synovial osteochondromatosis?

4. What gives rice bodies their low signal intensity on T2W images?

Exercise-Induced Rhabdomyolysis

1. High signal intensity changes in the muscle bodies of the quadriceps muscle group (except the rectus femoris).

2. Exercise-induced rhabdomyolysis. Squatting with heavy weights.

3. No, the signal intensity of the muscles will revert to normal within 1 to 2 weeks.

4. Pain and swelling.

References

Fleckenstein JL, Canby RC, Parkey RW, et al: Acute effects of exercise on MR imaging of skeletal muscle in normal volunteers. AJR Am J Roentgenol 151:231–237, 1988.

Shellock FG, Fukunaga T, Mink JH, Edgerton VR: Exertional muscle injury: Evaluation of concentric versus eccentric actions with serial MR imaging. Radiology 179:659–664, 1991.

Comments

An increase in both extracellular and intracellular water content normally occurs in muscles after exercise, the majority of the increase being extracellular. Magnetic resonance imaging is sensitive to the signal-intensity changes that occur in the muscle as a result of strenuous exercise. It is this alteration in T1 and T2 values that accounts for the increased signal intensity in the muscle on T2W images. A common clinical entity characterized by muscle pain several days after exercising, coined *delayed onset muscle soreness,* has been the focus of study. Clinically, a sensation of discomfort or pain occurs after muscular exertion. The pain increases in intensity in the first 24 hours after exercise, peaks after 24 to 72 hours, then subsides to normal after approximately 7 days. Shellock and colleagues demonstrated statistically significant increases in T2 relaxation times in biceps muscles in patients with delayed onset muscle soreness, with the highest mean measurements occurring between days 3 and 5. Prolongation of relaxation times on magnetic resonance images is considered to be primarily the result of accumulated edema, which develops shortly after severe exertional muscle injuries. Symptoms of pain and soreness, localized to the insertion sites of the exercised muscles, and discernible swelling and distention of the arms were maximal from days 3 to 10, correlating closely with peak T2 changes. Fleckenstein and associates also noted a high correlation among changes in muscle T2 relaxation time, pain, and elevation in serum creatine phosphokinase levels. This patient repeatedly squatted with 700-lb weights and had a serum creatine phosphokinase level of 211,000.

Rice Bodies (Juvenile Rheumatoid Arthritis)

1. Hypertrophied synovium, rice bodies, osteochondromatosis, and intra-articular fibrinous debris.

2. No hemosiderin deposition.

3. High signal intensity.

4. Fibrous tissue.

Reference

Chung C, Coley BD, Martin LC: Rice bodies in juvenile rheumatoid arthritis. AJR Am J Roentgenol 170:698–700, 1998.

Comments

Rice bodies, so named because of their similarity in appearance to grains of rice, are a nonspecific response to synovial inflammation. They are most commonly associated with synovial inflammatory arthritides, such as rheumatoid arthritis and juvenile rheumatoid arthritis, although rice bodies were originally described in association with tuberculous arthritis. Several etiologic theories have been suggested for the development of rice bodies, including microinfarction of the synovium with subsequent sloughing, encasement of entrapped cell in fibrinous exudates, and detachment of hypertrophied synovial villi. Radiographically, rice bodies are not distinctly evident, and patients present with either a mass or soft-tissue swelling. On magnetic resonance imaging, however, the findings are quite conspicuous, depicted as numerous tiny, well-defined nodules filling the affected joint and demonstrating intermediate signal intensity on T1W images and relatively lower signal intensity on T2W images. Administration of intravenous gadolinium reveals no enhancement of the rice bodies, although the adjacent synovium enhances brightly.

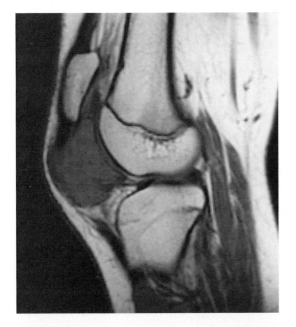
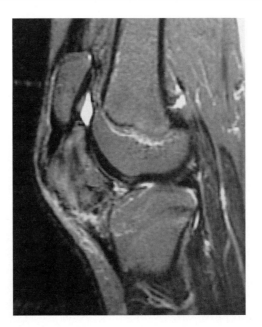

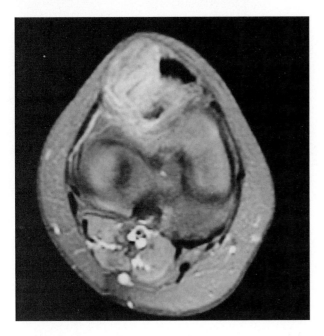

1. What should be done next?
2. Is a synovial sarcoma an intra-articular or an extra-articular neoplasm?
3. How frequently is calcification seen in synovial sarcomas?
4. When present, is erosive change in the bone a sign of benignity?

Synovial Sarcoma

1. Biopsy.

2. Both, but the majority are extra-articular.

3. Twenty to thirty percent of cases.

4. No, slow growth can cause erosive changes, but this does not equate with benignity.

Reference

Morton MJ, Berquist TH, McLeod RA, et al: MR imaging of synovial sarcoma. AJR Am J Roentgenol 156:337–340, 1991.

Comments

A synovial sarcoma is a highly malignant soft-tissue tumor, and, although it is rare, it constitutes the fourth most common soft-tissue neoplasm. It typically affects patients between the ages of 18 and 35 years, and it has no gender predilection. Most synovial sarcomas occur in the extremities, adjacent to a joint (knee, ankle, and foot are most common). However, fewer than 10% of tumors are intra-articular. These sarcomas may also arise from a tendon sheath. Clinically, patients present with painful soft-tissue swelling or mass. Although these tumors grow slowly, the prognosis is poor, with a 10-year survival rate of less than 30%.

Radiographically, a synovial sarcoma appears as a sharply marginated soft-tissue mass that may be lobulated and quite large. Calcifications within the tumor are evident in 20% to 30% of cases. Erosive changes in the adjacent bone and periosteal reactions may be seen in as many as 15% of cases. As the mass enlarges, more aggressive features may be noted. On magnetic resonance imaging, synovial sarcomas demonstrate low signal intensity on T1W images and heterogeneous to intense high signal intensity on T2W images. Fluid-fluid levels may occur secondary to hemorrhage. Administration of intravenous gadolinium demonstrates prominent enhancement, indicative of the hypervascular nature of the tumor. Treatment is surgical excision performed with a wide field. Recurrences happen at the initial site, and metastasis is generally to the lung.

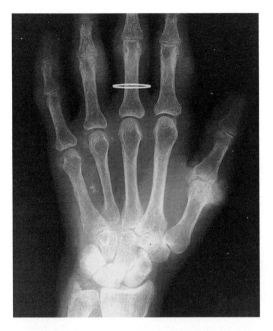
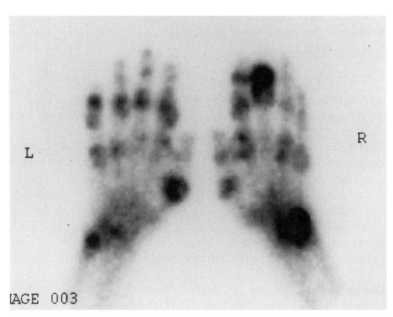

1. What is the most likely diagnosis?
2. What is the prevalence of chondrocalcinosis in the general population?
3. Is crystal deposition arthropathy common in the temporomandibular joints?
4. Do gouty tophi generally calcify?

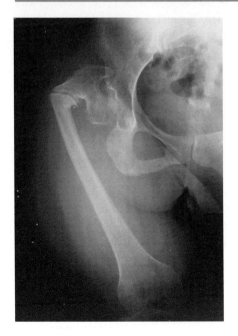

1. What are the main observations?
2. What do you call this entity?
3. Is this a unilateral or a bilateral condition?
4. Classification of this disorder is based on what observations?

Tophaceous Pseudogout

1. Tophaceous pseudogout.

2. About 0.9 per 1000.

3. No, it is rare.

4. No, only when there is also a disorder in calcium metabolism.

References

Huang GS, Bachmann D, Taylor JAM, et al: Calcium pyrophosphate dihydrate crystal deposition disease and pseudogout of the acromioclavicular joint: Radiographic and pathologic features. J Rheumatol 20:2077–2083, 1993.

Rivera-Sanfeliz G, Resnick D, Haghighi P, et al: Tophaceous pseudogout. Skeletal Radiol 25:699–701, 1996.

Comments

Calcium pyrophosphate dihydrate (CPPD) crystal deposition disease occurs with a frequency of 1 in 1000, with a prevalence that increases with age. The pseudogout syndrome is characterized by recurrent episodes of arthralgia caused by shedding of crystals into the synovial fluid of affected joints. The term *tophaceous pseudogout* was coined to describe massive periarticular soft-tissue crystal deposition in patients with pseudogout. The diagnosis is distinguished from gout by analysis of the synovial fluid, which reveals polarizable crystals of various shapes.

The main observation in this case of tophaceous pseudogout is the presence of tumorous periarticular soft-tissue calcifications that resemble the soft-tissue masses of tophaceous gout. In CPPD crystal deposition disease, these calcifications are common in the elbow, wrist, and pelvis. These calcifications may occur either in the joint (intra-articular deposits) or around the joint (periarticular deposits) and may be related to the deposition of both CPPD and hydroxyapatite crystals. Calcification of a gouty tophus is an unusual finding and usually reflects a coexisting abnormality of calcium metabolism. Otherwise, the calcific deposits in both diseases appear identical, with irregular or cloudlike radiodense masses localized to a periarticular distribution. The differential diagnosis of periarticular soft-tissue tumoral calcifications is extensive, but none produce the large soft-tissue masses presented in this case except for crystal-induced arthropathy and idiopathic tumoral calcinosis. Remember that the latter, however, does not involve the hands. The diagnosis is usually evident if other articulations reveal characteristic manifestations of CPPD arthropathy.

Proximal Femoral Focal Deficiency

1. Coxa vara deformity and focal dysgenesis of the proximal femur.

2. Proximal femoral focal deficiency (PFFD).

3. More than 90% of cases affect only one extremity.

4. Presence of the head of the femur, development of the acetabulum, length of femoral shortening, and relationship of the femur to the acetabulum at skeletal maturity.

Reference

Resnick D: Additional congenital or heritable anomalies and syndromes. In Diagnosis of Bone and Joint Disorders, 3rd ed. Philadelphia, WB Saunders, 1995, pp 4282–4285.

Comments

PFFD is a spectrum of congenital disorders that is characterized by segmental length discrepancy of the femur caused by defective formation of the proximal femur. The cause is unknown but occurs early in embryologic development, from a disturbance in either cellular nutrition or blood flow. There is an increased incidence in children of diabetic mothers. The majority of cases are unilateral. The segmental defect is usually isolated to the femur, although on rare occasions it has been reported to occur in association with tibial agenesis and aplasia of the cruciate ligaments of the knee.

There are four types. In type A, there is a varus deformity of the femoral neck, osseous connection between the components of the femur, and adequate development of the acetabulum. In type B, a pseudoarthrosis forms at the femoral neck, and there may be moderate dysplastic changes of the acetabulum. In type C, there is severe dysplasia of the acetabulum, a tapered proximal shaft, and variable connection between the femoral diaphysis and the poorly formed femoral head. In type D, the most severe deformity, there is absence of the acetabulum, enlargement of the obturator foramen, and absence of the proximal femur. Magnetic resonance imaging and ultrasound have been gaining preference over radiography and arthrography for early assessment of the condition because they allow imaging of nonossified cartilaginous structures.

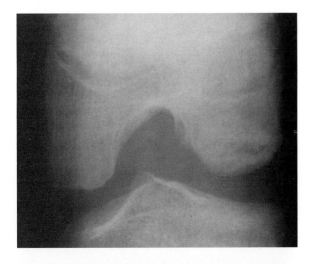

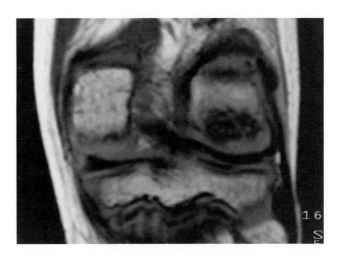

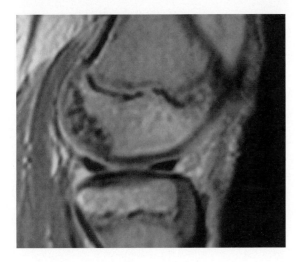

1. What is the diagnosis in this asymptomatic 10-year-old patient? What are the types depicted?
2. Where does this condition usually occur? What is its typical distribution?
3. Can this condition be recurrent?
4. What would you recommend as a follow-up?

Irregular Distal Femoral Epiphyseal Ossification

1. Irregularities of the ossification of the distal femoral epiphysis. Group 1 in the medial femoral condyle and group 3 in the lateral femoral condyle.

2. The posterior surface of the femoral condyles. Forty-four percent involve both medial and lateral femoral condyles, 44% affect the lateral femoral condyle only, and 12% affect the medial femoral condyle only.

3. Yes, it can occur in periods of rapid growth.

4. Nothing, but if you are pushed to do something, sequential radiographs would be expected to show improvement.

Reference

Caffey J, Madell SH, Royer C, Morales P: Ossification of the distal femoral epiphysis. J Bone Joint Surg Am 40:647–654, 1958.

Comments

Irregularities in the ossification of the distal femoral epiphyses are common in healthy children. Unfortunately, these variations in the pattern of ossification in the growing skeleton are often erroneously interpreted as evidence of disease. These irregularities are observed only in rapidly growing bones because the zones of proliferating cartilage and provisional calcifications are deeper than in slow-growing epiphysis. During accelerated growth, the orderly process of cartilage proliferation and provisional calcification may be disturbed, and foci of provisional calcification can appear beyond the main mass of calcified cartilage. As the invading osteoblasts replace the provisionally calcified cartilage by osseous trabeculation, the normal contour of the femoral epiphysis is restored.

Three groups of epiphyseal irregularities of the distal femur have been described. In group 1, there is localized roughening of the surface the distal epiphysis. In group 2, the marginal irregularities are larger and in the form of indentations. In group 3, the irregularities are similar to those of group 2, but there is also an independent island of bone within the crater, mimicking an osteochondral defect. Sequential radiographic examinations reveal eventual filling of the defect, usually within 2 years after the initial study. The incidence of the irregularities decreases with every decade of life, and they are seen in fewer than 10% of children older than 10 years.

Note: Page numbers followed by the letter f refer to figures.